ADVANCED POSTURE TAPING PROTOCOLS

AMERICAN POSTURE INSTITUTE

First printed edition: April 2021.

ISBN: 978-1-954665-00-2

Published by American Posture Institute

AMERICAN POSTURE INSTITUTE
151 San Francisco Street
San Juan, Puerto Rico, 00901, US
www.americanpostureinstitute.com

Dedication

This book is dedicated to the American Posture
Institute community of Posture Experts.
Your success is our priority.

Editor's Preface

The purpose of this book is to provide practitioners with a practical understanding of how to apply and utilize Posture Tape for patient and client management. At the American Posture Institute we provide healthcare professionals with advanced education in posture and posture related topics. *Advanced Posture Taping* serves the purpose of helping healthcare providers implement Posture Taping protocols as part of their overall patient management strategy.

I was encouraged to write this book after struggling to understand if Posture Tape was actually beneficial or not for patient care. After performing research and testing these systems I discovered that Posture Tape, when applied correctly can be highly beneficial for patients, and a great tool for practitioners to have in their clinical tool belts.

My name is Dr. Krista Burns, founder of the American Posture Institute and dual doctorate with a clinical doctorate degree in chiropractic and an educational doctorate degree in health administration with an emphasis in health policy. As a practitioner and educator I have a profound interest in posture, neurology, and human physiology.

I have had the great honor of teaching thousands of healthcare professionals from across the world. I am a TEDx Speaker, have spoken at the World Congress of Falls and Postural Stability, and have had the privilege of speaking for universities and professional organizations in 12 countries across 4 continents. My work has been featured in the media including ABC, NBC, CBS, and Fox News Radio affiliates.

At the American Posture Institute we provide post-graduate online learning programs in Structural Postural Correction, Brain Based Postural Correction, Postural Ergonomics, and Pediatric Postural Correction. We also have advanced trainings in ancillary therapies such as *Advanced Posture Taping*.

We are on a mission to reverse postural decline in the digital age. At the American Posture Institute we believe that it is *Posture by Design, Not by Circumstance.* With postural correction and posture habit re-education patients can rise above the conditions of their environment and stand tall with proper posture.

We are committed to this mission. By training healthcare professionals to implement postural correction solutions with their patients the American Posture Institute has made a global impact.

By reading *Advanced Posture Taping* you will learn practical application of how to use Posture Tape for improved proprioception, pain management, and posture habit re-education. It is recommended to implement Posture Taping protocols with a complete postural correction system.

This book is designed for practitioners who want to understand why Posture Tape works, how to determine what protocol to apply, and how to apply Posture Tape for maximal benefit. This is for you if you are dedicated to advanced learning for practical application.

This book is not intended to be medical advice. It is the personal responsibility of the practitioner applying the Posture Tape to know their local regulations and licensure for proper application within their specialty. It is not the liability of the American Posture Institute. Each practitioner and patient is liable for his or her own health and for the application of treatments.

For instructional videos and demonstrations of how to apply Posture Tape, please join us for the *Advanced Posture Taping* online course. To learn more about the American Posture Institute and how you can integrate postural correction systems, visit us at <u>AmericanPostureInstitute.com</u>.

At the American Posture Institute we have high integrity for posture education. We value you, our community of Posture Expert Professionals. We live by our #1 core value that *Your Success is Our Priority.*

TABLE OF CONTENTS

CHAPTER 1

THEORY AND PRINCIPLES OF POSTURE TAPING

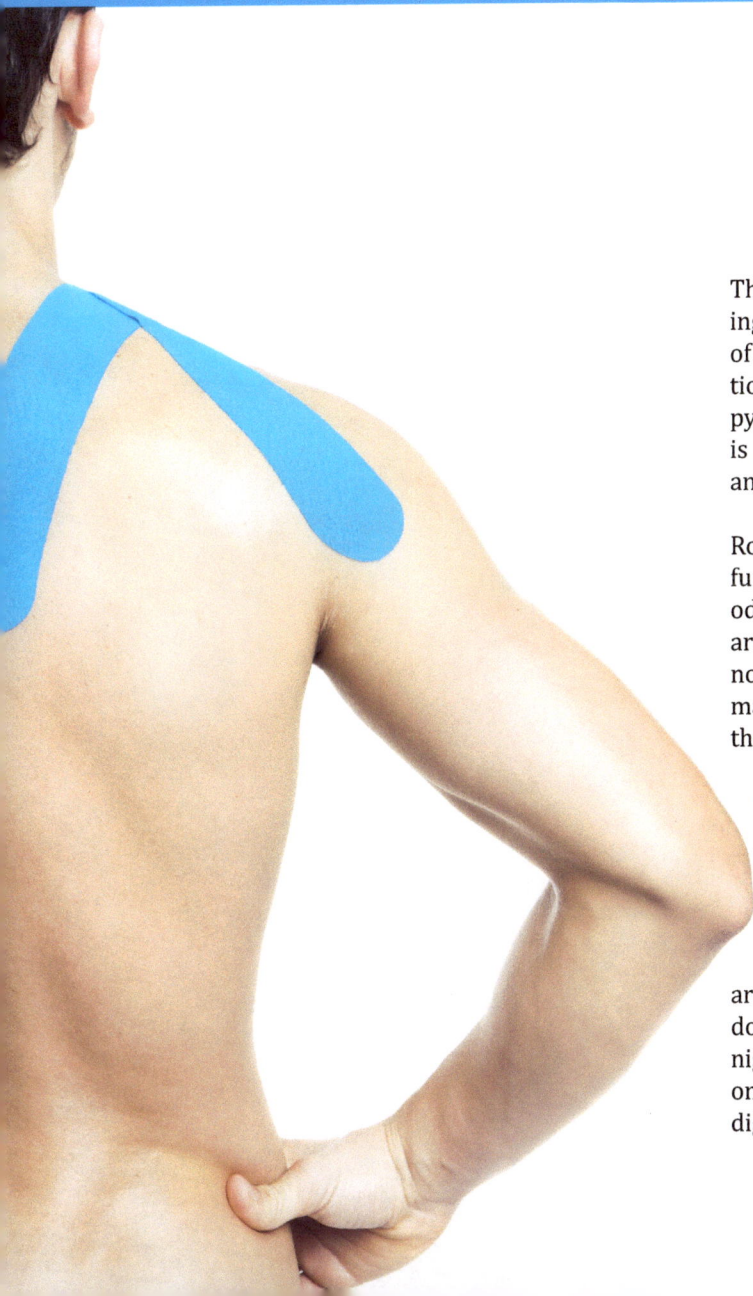

The utilization of Kinesio Tape has become increasingly popular in recent years. Although the utilization of traditional taping methods to restrict range of motion have been used for a long time in physiotherapy, the utilization of Kinesio Tape is rather new and is gaining popularity among healthcare practitioners and patients alike.

Kinesio Tape, along with other brands such as Rock Tape, K Tape, and others are all considered functional tapes. Unlike the traditional taping methods that restrict range of motion, used when patients are hypermobile or instable, functional taping does not restrict range of motion. Functional taping has many different uses, which we will explain in detail throughout this course.

Functional taping has gained popularity in recent years. One of the primary reasons for increased awareness of functional taping is that many famous athletes utilize the tape, and spectators took notice of the neon colored tapes in non-traditional patterns on athlete's bodies. It went from traditional white ankle tape to neon pink Y-straps around the shoulder with blue fan-shaped strips down the leg. Famous athletes, what seemed like over night, were suddenly wearing this new tape. Everyone took notice. From here the Functional Tape paradigm exploded.

Recent movements in healthcare and exercise protocols have also noted the importance of "Function," making "Function" a new buzzword among patients and healthcare professionals. From functional movements, functional patterns, functional training, functional exercise protocols, we now have Functional Tape. A popular mindset shift from "reactive care" to "functional care" has become apparent, and the utilization of Kinesio Tape fits appropriately within this paradigm, benefitting your top athletes and your average 40 hour a week day job patients.

Kinesio Tape has gained its popularity on this premise of improved function. While improving function, the tape is also effective for postural correction when utilized as an ancillary component of a complete posture correction protocol.

At the American Posture Institute, we utilize and encourage Posture Experts to use a three-component model to achieve complete postural correction. This model includes spinal alignment, posture rehabilitation, and posture habit re-education as a 360-degree approach to the complete correction of postural distortion patterns that limiting human function.

Posture Taping, when utilized in this model fits within the category of Posture Habit Re-Education. The purpose of posture habit re-education is to re-educate common habits that cause postural collapse in patients' daily lives. Common examples of poor postural habits are sleeping face down, slouching while sitting, hunching the neck forward while looking at your computer screen... so many of our patients are guilty of these seemingly small bad habits. What they don't realize is that overtime, these repetitive postural habits are shaping their human physiology.

IDEAL POSTURAL PRESENTATION

Before we continue our discussion of poor posture habits and postural distortion patterns. Let's consider what healthy, ideal posture is. Healthy postural presentation is characterized as the ability to resist gravity in an efficient, upright position. Ideal posture is symmetrically balanced bilaterally, and from the anterior to the posterior aspect in relation to the patient's center of gravity.

Patients with ideal postural design have strong core musculature that supports the proper alignment of the spine and the pelvis. The postural muscles and the joints among the kinetic chain of movement have accurate recruitment patterns and full range of motion. Agonist and antagonist muscle groups fire and stabilize together in synchrony. The connective tissue is fluid, not tightly bound into contracture. The patient has strong postural muscles and mobile joints, so that when they perform dynamic movements they don't have postural collapse. The brain, cerebellum, and the body produce coordinated and controlled movements. Their body is in proper alignment and they have developed postural fitness to maintain it.

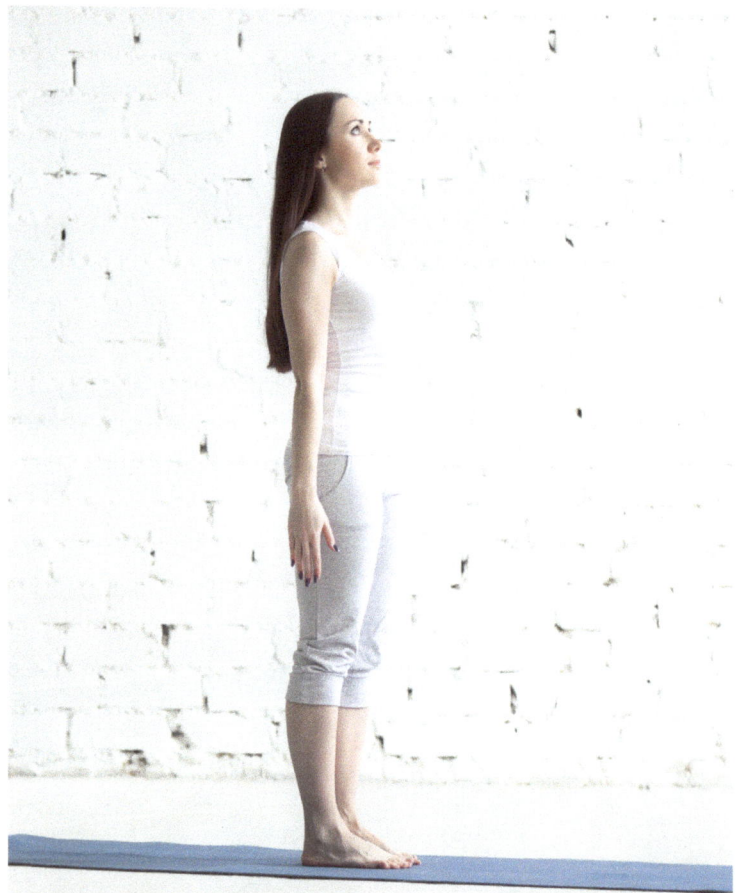

When viewing patients from the anterior pers-pective, you would see the following clinical findings with ideal posture:

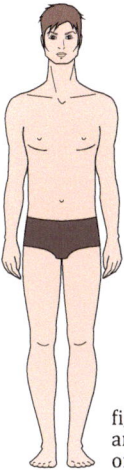

figure 1-2:
anterior view
of a male patient

ANTERIOR VIEW OF THE PATIENT:

- **Head:** Neutral position (no lateral flexion or rotation)
- **Eyes:** Parallel to the horizon
- **Ears:** Level with one another bilaterally
- **Chin:** Centered (not rotated to one side)
- **Shoulders:** Level bilaterally (not elevated or depressed), even muscular development, and pulled back (not rotated forward)
- **Arms:** Neutral position, at even lengths, palms toward the lateral aspect of the body with the thumbs pointed forward
- **Pelvis:** Level, both anterior superior iliac spines and pelvic crests are in the same transverse plane
- **Hip Joints:** Neutral position (no abduction or adduction, or flexion or extension)
- **Patellae:** Level bilaterally, pointed forward
- **Feet:** Parallel with slight out-toeing. The medialmalleoli are in the same vertical plane (no pro-nation or supination is present)

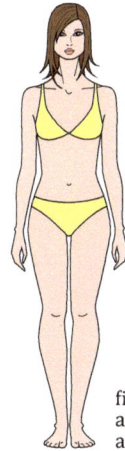

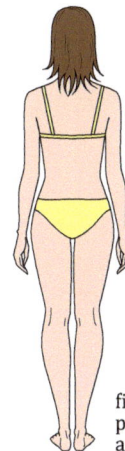

figure 1-2:
anterior view of
a female patient

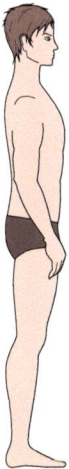

From the lateral perspective, you would expect to see the follow-ing findings with ideal posture:

figure 1-3:
lateral view
of a male patient

LATERAL VIEW OF THE PATIENT:

- **Head:** Neutral position (no flexion or extension)
- **Eyes:** Parallel to the horizon
- **Ear:** Aligned over the shoulder
- **Cervical Spine:** Normal curve with slight anterior convexity
- **Thoracic Spine:** Normal curve with slight posterior convexity
- **Shoulders:** Back (not rotated forward), aligned over the hips
- **Arms:** Neutral position, at even lengths, palms toward the lateral aspect of the body with the thumbs pointed forward
- **Lumbar Spine:** Normal curve with slight anterior convexity
- **Pelvis:** Neutral position, the anterior superior iliac spineis in the same vertical plane as the pubic symphisis
- **Hip Joint:** Neutral position, neither extended or flexed
- **Knee:** Neutral position, neither extended or flexed
- **Ankle:** Neutral position, leg is vertical and at a right angle to the sole of the foot
- **Feet:** Pointed forward

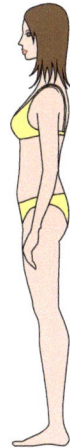

figure 1-4:
lateral view of
a female patient

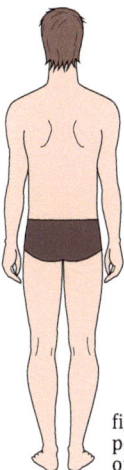

And from the posterior aspect of the patient, you would expect to see the following features:

figure 1-5:
posterior view
of a male patient

POSTERIOR VIEW OF THE PATIENT:

- **Head:** Neutral position (no lateral flexion or rotation)
- **Ears:** Level with one another bilaterally
- **Shoulders:** Level bilaterally (not elevated or depressed), even muscular development, and pulled back (not rotated forward)
- **Scapulae:** Medial borders are parallel and about 4 inches apart
- **Arms:** Neutral position, at even lengths, palms toward the lateral aspect of the body
- **Thoracic Spine:** No lateral deviation
- **Pelvis:** Level, both posterior superior iliac spines and pelvic crests are in the same transverse plane
- **Hip Joints:** Neutral position (no abduction or adduction, or flexion or extension)
- **Achilles' Tendons:** Parallel bilaterally (no supination or pronation)
- **Feet:** Parallel with slight out-toeing. The medial malleoli are in the same vertical plane (no pronation or supination is present)

figure 1-6:
posterior view of
a female patient

Any deviation from "ideal" posture would be considered a postural distortion. Multiple posture distortions noted throughout the Posture System of the body are considered postural distortion patterns.

The most common postural distortion patterns that patients present with while standing are forward head posture, a hyperkyphotic-lordotic spinal pre-sentation, anterior pelvic tilt, pelvic unleveling, and pronation of the feet.

Forward head posture is defined by Sylva et al. (2009) as "the protrusion of the head in the sagittal plane so that the head is placed anterior to the trunk." Raine and Twomey (1997) suggest that forward head posture is the result of an extended cervical spine, protracted shoulder girdles, and a hyperkyphotic thoracic spine. When a patient presents with forward head posture, their eyes seek eye level with the horizon causing the cervical spine to go into extension. When the cervical spine is extended, there is approximation of the occiput and C7.

Kyphotic-lordotic spinal presentation is an increased posterior curve of the thoracic spine with an increased anterior curve of the lumbar spine. With this common postural distortion pattern, patients present with medial rotation of the shoulders. The thoracic spine demonstrates increased flexion, or kyphosis. With an increased lordosis, or hyperextension of the lumbar spine, the pelvis tilts anteriorly and the hip joints are flexed.

Anterior pelvic tilt occurs as the pelvis tilts forward, and can be viewed from the lateral aspect of the patient. Anterior pelvic tilt is characterized by tight hip flexors and lumbar paraspinal musculature, and weakened hip extensors such as the gluteus maximus and the hamstrings as well as weak rectus abominis muscles.

Pelvic unleveling is viewed anteriorly and/or posteriorly by evaluating the level of the iliac spines and the pelvic crests anteriorly, and by evaluating the level of the pelvic crests, the iliac spines, and the sacroiliac joints posteriorly. With pelvic unleveling, there is a visual high hip with an ipsilateral visual leg length discrepancy, which can easily be seen as the patient is lying prone or supine.

Foot pronation is the most common postural distortion pattern of the foot. It is most commonly bilateral, however, if not bilateral it is more commonly associated with the long leg. Pronation is characterized as abduction, dorsal flexion, and eversion of the foot. Visual postural analyses demonstrate a prominent ankle on the inside and a sunken one on the outside with weight distribution on the medial border of the foot.

While seated, patients most commonly present with forward head posture, hyperkyphosis of the thoracic spine, and anterior translation of the pelvis with posterior pelvic tilt.

Certified Posture Experts are highly trained in performing complete postural analyses to determine for the presence of postural distortion patterns. They do a complete posture examination along with the utilization of Posture Imaging to determine exactly where postural distortion patterns are present.

Once the postural distortion patterns have been detected and analyzed, the Posture Expert then creates a treatment plan including the 3 component-postural correction system for complete postural correction. A full explanation of each of these components, including correction modalities are included in the Certified Posture Expert online course.

For purposes of this advanced course in Posture Taping, we will be discussing in detail the third component of the complete postural correction system, which is posture habit re-education.

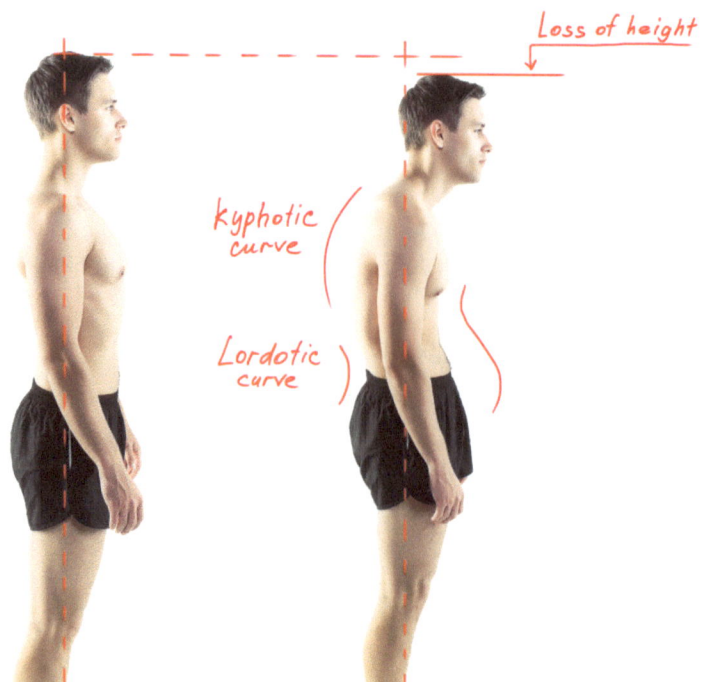

POSTURE HABIT RE-EDUCATION

"Habits are defined as actions that are triggered automatically in response to contextual cues that have been associated with their performance" (Neal et al., 2012). Habits are cognitively efficient actions because the automation of common actions frees mental resources for other tasks. However, the process of creating new habits, or healthy habits, is a mindful process.

Gardner et al. (2012) explains the relevance of habit-formation principles in achieving desired health outcomes. They suggest the formation of new habits is a simple formula. It may not be easy to adhere to, this requires motivation and mindful dedication in achieving the outcome, but the formula itself is simple.

To create a new habit Gardner et al. (2012) suggests, repeat an action consistently in the same context. The habit formation attempt begins at the 'initiation phase', during which the new behavior and the context in which it will be done are selected. Automaticity develops in the subsequent 'learning phase', during which the behavior is repeated in the chosen context to strengthen the context-behavior association. Habit-formation culminates in the 'stability phase', at which the habit has formed and its strength has plateaued, so that it persists over time with minimal effort (Gardner et al., 2012).

The purpose of re-educating postural habits is for intentional postural awareness and mindfulness of the body in its surrounding environment. Through posture habit re-education, the patient creates new neural pathways that support proper postural design. The goal of posture habit re-education is to retrain the postural patterns of the body through neuromuscular re-education.

A focus on posture habit re-education should be performed daily to create efficient muscle memory sequences. Posture habit re-education is fundamental for

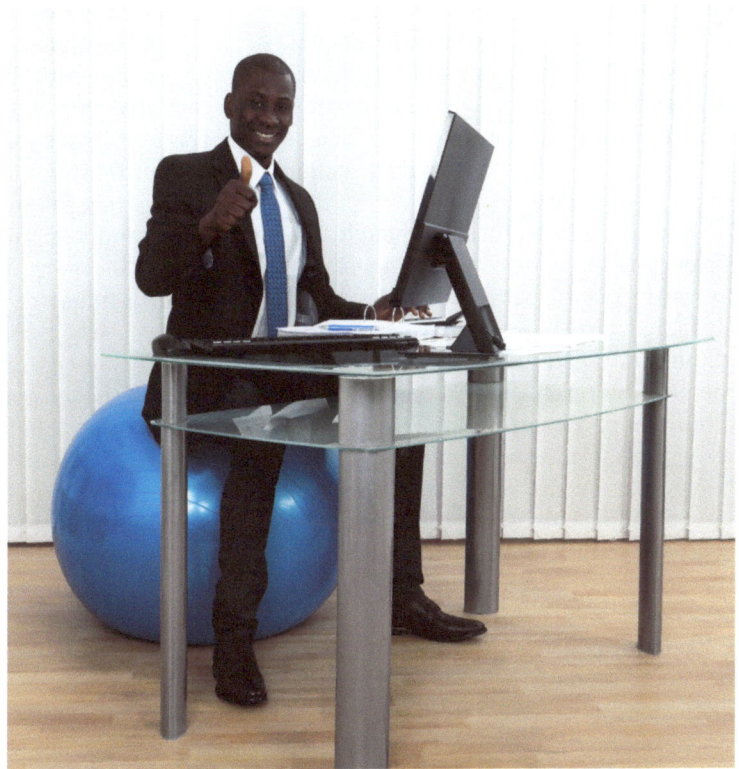

long-term postural changes to be maintained. In order to change habits, it requires a commitment to a change in lifestyle. If the patient is not committed, it will be much more difficult, or even impossible to change their postural habits.

Mindfulness is postural awareness. At any given moment we are either elongating and opening the posture system or shortening and compressing it. For long-term postural correction, the patient needs to be mindful and intentional with their movements. They should perform movements that work with the natural design of the body, not against it. To create mindfulness, the patient should utilize "posture reminders."

A posture reminder can be a sticker that they place in the areas where they spend the most amount of time, or it could be an alarm set on the clock to go off multiple times throughout the day, or even a bracelet that the patient wears. When the patient sees the posture reminder they will be prompted to be mindful of their bodily position and make necessary corrections for proper posture. For example, if the patient is at their desk at work and they see their posture sticker at their computer, they will be reminded to check their posture. This brings posture back into their consciousness mind so they can modify their working posture in that moment if necessary. Posture reminders help patients succeed in changing their posture.

Posture Taping can be utilized as a posture reminder to remind the patient to maintain proper posture. With the tape on, the patient can actually feel when they have proper posture and when they do not. The patient has a visual and kinesthetic relationship with the tape that makes it a highly effective posture reminder as a part of their complete postural correction treatment plan.

Neural plasticity occurs though consistency with posture habit re-education to create neural pathways that support sustained postural health. When beginning to create new habits, or muscle memory patterns, engage the conscious mind. There are many different ways of engaging the conscious mind to change habits that are discussed in psychosocial literature journals. Kelly et al. (1991) discusses the dimensions of health beliefs that influence patients in making changes to their lifestyle habits. The most significant dimensions of health that influence the motivation for patients to make lifestyle changes include the perceived risk of continuing the lifestyle behavior that should be changed, the benefit of changing the lifestyle behavior, the social support that the patient receives from their family, friends, and colleagues, and the magnitude of self-efficacy that the patient will achieve when they change that lifestyle habit.

Each of these dimensions is important in lasting habit changes. The two dimensions that were demonstrated by Kelly et al. (1991) to have the most profound affect on motivation for changing lifestyle habits are the perceived benefits that the patient will experience with the changed habit and the magnitude of self-efficacy that they will achieve. In addition to these factors, extrinsic rewards are also shown to increase patients' level of motivation in making lifestyle changes.

It is very important to consider the psychosocial aspect of habit creation, and utilize this information when conversing with patients. Recognize what motivates your patients, and discuss the benefits of having proper posture with them. Skip the features of the tape when communicating with your patients. For example, they don't need to know who invented Kinesio Tape and the features of the tension limits. What they DO need to know is the benefit that they will receive from wearing the Posture Tape, and how it will assist them in their overall goal of posture habit transformations to support proper postural design during daily activities and occupational activities.

As Teutsch (2003) explains, effective healthcare encompasses the art of human interaction. The challenges of doctor to patient communication include understanding how the patient's condition is affecting their quality of life, and then empowering the patient to make appropriate choices on personal health issues. The ability to communicate effectively is crucial to bringing the benefits of postural correction to patients, and is important to the professional satisfaction that patients get from doctor to patient interactions.

Once the need for posture habit re-education is determined and the patient is motivated to take action, then be ready to suggest successful posture habit interventions to re-educate their postural patterns.

Verplanken and Wood (2006) suggest that successful habit change interventions involve disrupting the environmental factors that automatically cue habit performance. Common cues for postural collapse are sitting in front of a computer, texting, or sitting on the couch. If you know that your patients experience postural collapse while performing these two activities, teach them to disrupt old environmental cues that they associate with poor posture and establish new cues that they associate with mindful posture. The implementation of new habit cues can be simple, as for example the utilization of posture stickers in the places where your patients experience postural collapse, or wearing Posture Tape. These new cues will stimulate conscious mindfulness of their posture.

Consistent repetition of these new postural habits is a process of associative learning in which the action being activated upon is in context with sequential exposure to the cues, in this case Posture Reminders or Posture Tape. Once initiation of the action is 'transferred' to external cues, dependence on conscious attention or motivational processes is reduced. As this occurs habits are likely to persist even after conscious motivation or interest dissipates.

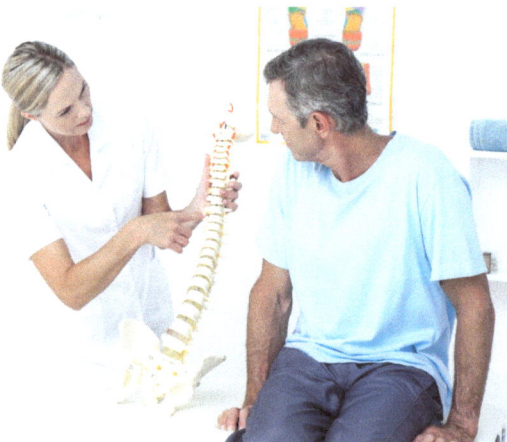

PATIENT COMPLIANCE TO LIFESTYLE CHANGES

In healthcare, the most commonly used definition of compliance is "patient's behaviors (in terms of taking medication, following diets, or executing lifestyle changes) coincide with healthcare providers' recommendations for health and medical advice" (Sackett, 1976). Therapeutic non-compliance, therefore, occurs when a patient's lifestyle behaviors lack congruence with the recommendations of their healthcare provider.

To genuinely impact your patients' health, patient compliance issues are a serious consideration that should be addressed by Posture Experts. According to DiMatteo (1995) compliance with lifestyle changes is the lowest category of compliance, at only 20%–30% compliance.

What are the primary factors contributing to patient non-compliance? Jin et al. (2008) evaluated the primary factors affecting patients' therapeutic compliance. The main factor attributing to patient non-compliance was the patient's perception of side effects or pain when using the therapy for a long duration. Posture Experts can easily address this factor of non-compliance by communicating with their patients each time a therapy is recommended – both for posture habit re-education and for posture rehabilitation. Also, avoid long durations when discussing objectives with patients, give them short-term recommendations. Give them small goals to achieve, or with the example of Posture Taping, tell the patient you want to see how they feel at the next visit. Long duration goals are more abstract to patients and they can't see the immediate benefit of complying to your advice. Give them short-term objectives to keep them stimulated and improve patient compliance.

The second factor contributing to patient non-compliance is related to patient satisfaction of the healthcare facility and accessibility (Jin et al., 2008). If patients experience long wait times, or find it difficult to reach the healthcare facility, they are shown to be less compliant. This can be avoided by having efficient procedures in which the patient is not treated as a number, they are taken care of, and the procedures in your office support clinically precise and efficient work. If a patient has to wait 30 minutes for a 3-minute application of Posture Tape, their satisfaction will drop, and likely affect their compliance.

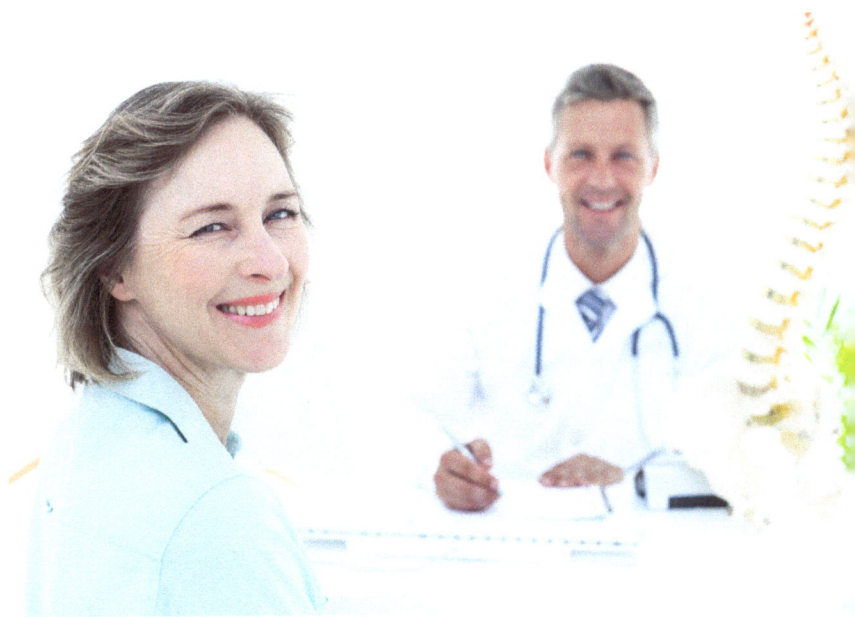

The third factor contributing to non-compliance is related to chronicity. Acute patients have better compliance than chronic patients (Jin et al., 2008). When dealing with chronic patients, take this into consideration. Utilize the communication strategies that we just discussed, and help them see the benefits of your treatment. They don't need all of the features, they just need you to provide them with hope. They need to see the benefit they will receive from complete posture correction.

Posture Tape, when applied correctly and when effectively communicated to the patient, should be great for patient compliance. Posture Tape is an "easy" therapy for the patient. They simply wear it, receive therapeutic benefit, and train their bodies to sustain the proper position through conscious posture habit re-education.

Functional tapes are acrylic tape, not latex, meaning that there is less skin irritation so patients are more likely to leave it connected to the skin. The 100% cotton fibers allow for evaporation and quicker drying. This allows Kinesio tape to be worn in the shower or pool without having to be reapplied. Kinesio tape can be applied to virtually any muscle or joint in the body, and is recommended for usage for 3-4 days after the initial application. Patients in our office also report wearing the tape before it came off for up to 7-day intervals. Plus, they can perform all of their normal activities with the tape on.

The elimination of perspiration, freedom of motion and a smooth feeling of the tape are particular properties of Functional tape that have been shown to be desirable to athletes (Huang et al., 2011). The benefits far outweigh the effort necessary of wearing the Posture Tape for all populations of patients.

If patients are non-compliant to other aspects of their complete postural correction treatment plan, Posture Taping is a good therapy to use that is simple for the patient to be compliant to. Address the non-compliance issues that could be preventing your patients from achieving optimal postural correction and offer them solutions that meet their personal objectives, occupation, and lifestyle.

Communicate to patients in words that they understand, and strive to meet their patient centered needs. According to Detsky (2011), the highest priorities for patients worldwide are to achieve relief from symptoms, to have symptom relief within a timely manner, and to feel as though their healthcare provider was kind and gave them hope and certainty.

Give your patients safe opportunities to continue doing postural correction treatment in your clinic. Make it about them, and give them what they want based upon your clinical assessment. When you meet their needs, patient compliance for patient's achieving their desired healthcare results is greatly increased.

WHAT IS FUNCTIONAL TAPE AND HOW DOES IT WORK?

What is Functional Tape and how does it work? A point of clarification is necessary when answering the questions "What is Functional Tape, and how does it work?" Unless otherwise specified, when discussing Functional tape and Posture Tape we are referring to applications of Kinesio Tape, which is one of the many brands available for Functional Tape. In Module 3 we will discuss the different brands in a product review so that you can find the desired tape for your clinic and to utilize with your patients.

Functional tape differs greatly from traditional taping methods that have been used as part of the PRICE protocol. The acronym PRICE refers to Protection, Rest, Ice, Compression, and Elevation. Traditional, restrictive tape is utilized for compression of the injured tissue to prevent range of motion as part of the PRICE protocol.

As this type of tape is supportive and the objective is to reduce range of motion, traditional taping methods are utilized specifically for patients who present with hypermobility. For example, there are patients who have hypermobile ankles and report frequently rolling their ankles and suffering from recurrent sprains. When patients present with similar case presentations of hypermobility, it is recommended to use restrictive, rigid tape to prevent recurrent injury.

Restrictive taping is widely used in the field of rehabilitation as both a means of treatment and prevention of sports--related injuries. The essential function of rigid tape is to provide support during movement. The most commonly used restrictive tape applications are done with non--stretch tape with the rationale of providing protection and support to a joint or a muscle (Thelen et al., 2008).

In recent years, the use of Kinesio Tape has become increasingly popular. Kinesio tape, invented by Kenzo Kase in 1996, is a new application of adhesive taping. It is a thin and elastic tape, which has the capability of being stretched up to 120-140% of its original length, making it quite elastic and resulting in less mechanism constraints, when compared with traditional tape.

Kinesio tape was designed to mimic the qualities of human skin with roughly the same thickness as the epidermis layer of the skin. The elasticity of Kinesio Tape conforms to the body, allowing for movement. The tape is latex-free, very thin, and stretches in the longitudinal plane.

Kase et al. (1996) have proposed several benefits of the utilization of Kinesio Tape. Results vary depending on the amount of stretch applied to the tape and to the skin during application.

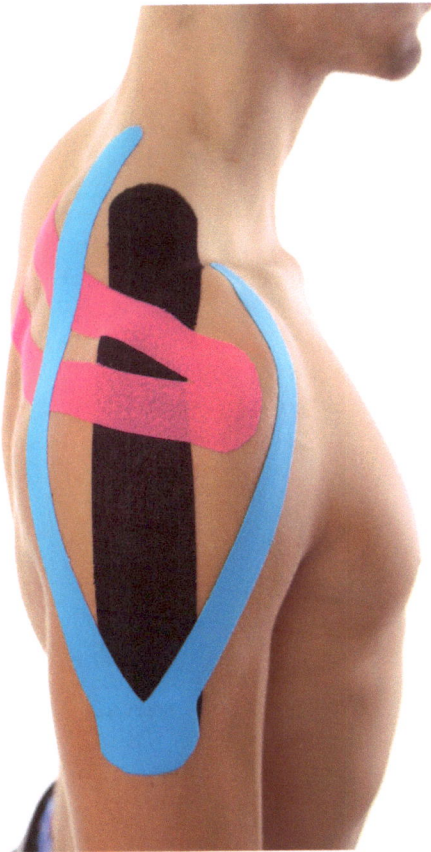

PROPOSED BENEFITS OF KINESIO TAPE:
(Kase et al., 1996)

1. To provide a positional stimulus through the skin
2. To align fascial tissues
3. To create more space by lifting fascia and soft tissue above area of pain/inflammation
4. To provide sensory stimulation to assist or limit motion
5. To assist in the removal of edema by directing exudates toward a lymph duct. KT is unique in several respects when compared to most commercial brands of tape. It is latex free and the adhesive is 100% acrylic and heat activated.

According to Huang et al. (2011) the beneficial effects of Functional Tape include physical corrections, fascia relaxation, space recuperation, ligament and tendon support, movement rectification and lymphatic fluid circulation. Strachan and Sandstrom (2015) propose that kinesio tape offloads fascia of injured tissues to decrease pain while facilitating an up-regulation of neurological control.

The two main theories proposed to explain the reported functional effects of Kinesio Tape are increased blood and lymphatic fluid circulation in the taped area due to a lifting effect, which creates a wider space between the skin and the muscle and interstitial space (Halseth et al., 2004). An additional theory is that Kinesio tape may apply pressure or continual stretching of the skin within the taped area, and this external activation of cutaneous mechanoreceptors would activate modulatory mechanisms within the central nervous system demonstrated as an increase in muscle excitability and proprioception (Gomez-Soriano, 2013).

EVIDENCE-BASED CLINICAL PROTOCOL

Let's have a discussion about the evidence supporting Kinesio Taping protocols. Some clinicians say that there is no research supporting the clinical effectiveness of Kinesio Tape. This statement, I would argue is not true. There are multiple studies demonstrating the clinical efficacy of Kinesio Tape, however, there are also multiple studies demonstrating that the changes seen with Kinesio Tape are minimal and not clinically significant.

As a modern-day healthcare practitioner, it is necessary to follow evidence-based guidelines. However, don't discredit the anecdotal clinical data that you are collecting each day from the patients in your office. Listen to their responses, see if your patients want and like Posture Tape, and then look for objective changes demonstrating the need for continued care.

According to Nakajima and Baldridge (2013), the inconsistency among studies may be attributed to how the experiments were conducted. For example, functional tape may have a different effect on eccentric muscle contraction and concentric muscle contraction. Also, the amount of tension applied to the tape will have an affect on the outcomes of the study.

For example, Vithoulk and colleagues compared the effect of Kinesio Tape on healthy female individuals on peak muscle torque of the dominant knee extensors by using isokinetic dynamometer for concentric and eccentric strength. Results indicated a statistically significant increase in eccentric isokinetic exercise of the quadriceps muscle under the Kinesio tape condition compared to the no-tape and sham condition. However, no difference was found for concentric muscle strength. Vercelli and colleagues only examined concentric muscle strength and did not find any effects related to Kinesio tape.

It has also been shown that Functional Taping makes more of an impact on compromised tissue. Thedon et al conducted a study to evaluate body sway in individuals with and without tape. They found that the tape showed very little change in the uncompromised condition, but when the subjects were fatigued, the tape provided an added stimulatory effect to the skin helping to compensate for the loss of information fed to the brain from the muscles and joints. For the pain and performance community, this study provides insight into an "auxiliary" system, such as the skin, to augment treatment and training outcomes (Trotter, 2013).

It is important to recognize that Functional Taping is a new concept, and research on this topic is only a few years old. More research is necessary to make definitive conclusions about the effectiveness of Kinesio Tape. As of now, you are challenged, as a Practitioner to note what clinical findings your patients are experiencing in your office.

This is an ancillary modality that should be used if you see clinical improvements with your patients and if patients are satisfied with it. From our perspective, at the American Posture Institute,

Posture Taping is an effective mode of ancillary posture correction and is a useful posture habit re-education strategy that our patients respond favorably to.

A literature review will be provided in Module 2. In Module 2 we will discuss each quadrant of the Posture System, and how Functional Tape can be effective for therapeutic relief for your patients. We will also discuss the research of Posture Taping for the most common postural distortions present in each posture quadrant of the body.

The limited information on Functional Tape application suggests improved function, pain, stability, and proprioception in pediatrics and patients with acute patellar dislocation, stroke, ankle pain, shoulder pain, and trunk dysfunction (Thelen et al., 2008). Further information will be explored on each of these case presentations in Module 2 when we discuss the application of Posture Tape for each of the posture quadrants of the Posture System.

POSTURE TAPING AND ITS RELATION TO THE POSTURE SYSTEM

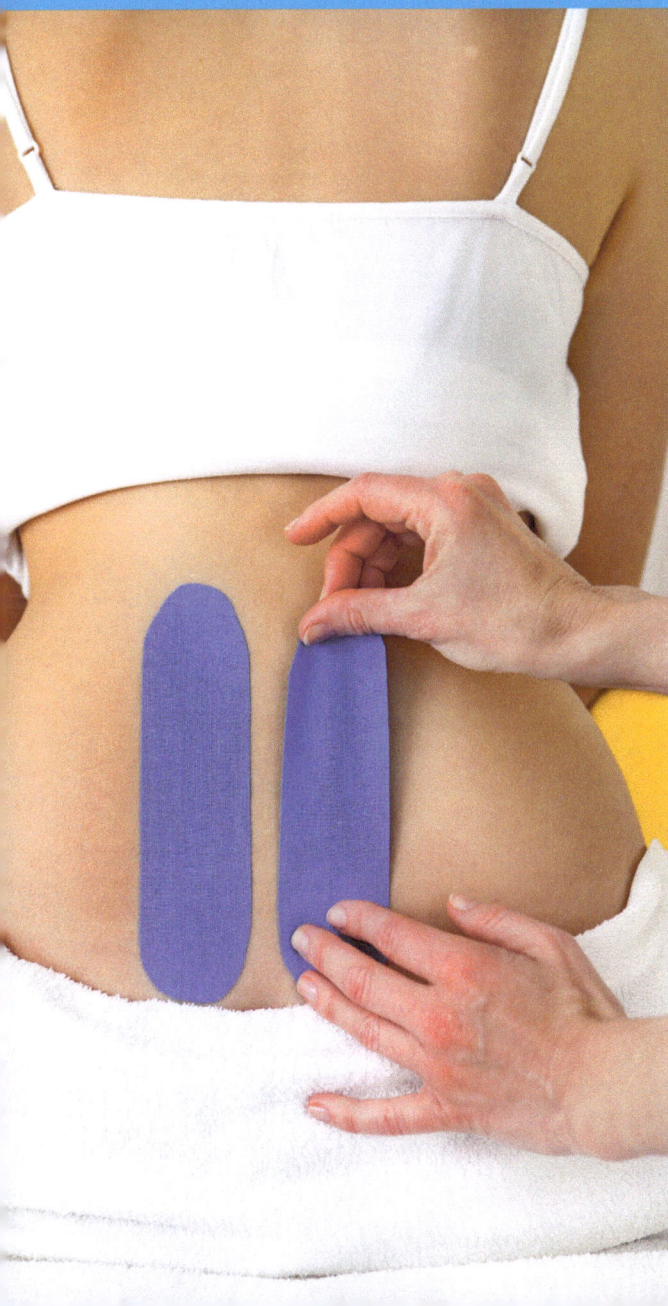

In Module 1 you learned the theories and principles of what Functional Tape is, and the rationale of why you would consider using it with your patients. We discussed how Functional Taping is an effective strategy in terms of patient compliance when communicated correctly to the patient. The therapeutic and functional benefits of utilizing Functional Tape should greatly outweigh the effort required by the patient. This is important for patient satisfaction and compliance with your recommendations.

In Module 2 we will provide a literature review pertinent to the therapeutic, structural, and functional benefits of Functional Taping protocols for each of the posture quadrants within the Posture System. We will present both sides of the research allowing you to make accurate clinical decisions for the utilization of Functional Tape applications for your patients.

The application of Functional Tape is to be utilized at the discretion of the Posture Expert. There are many different reasons why, and ways how to use functional tape within your clinic, all of which we will discuss in greater detail in Modules 3 and 4. When determining whether or not to use Functional Tape for purposes of posture or therapeutic relief, think first what the desired clinical objective is, then make your clinical decision based upon this desired result.

Functional tape is not utilized initially for the care of acute injuries, unless the purpose of the application is to assist in controlling edema or bruising, or to reduce muscle spasms. Acute injuries, such as an ankle sprain will likely need stabilizing tape initially. However, as the patient enters the rehabilitation phase of the injury, Functional tape can be applied with other modalities to increase function while minimizing pain and to improve strength, muscle firing, and coordination.

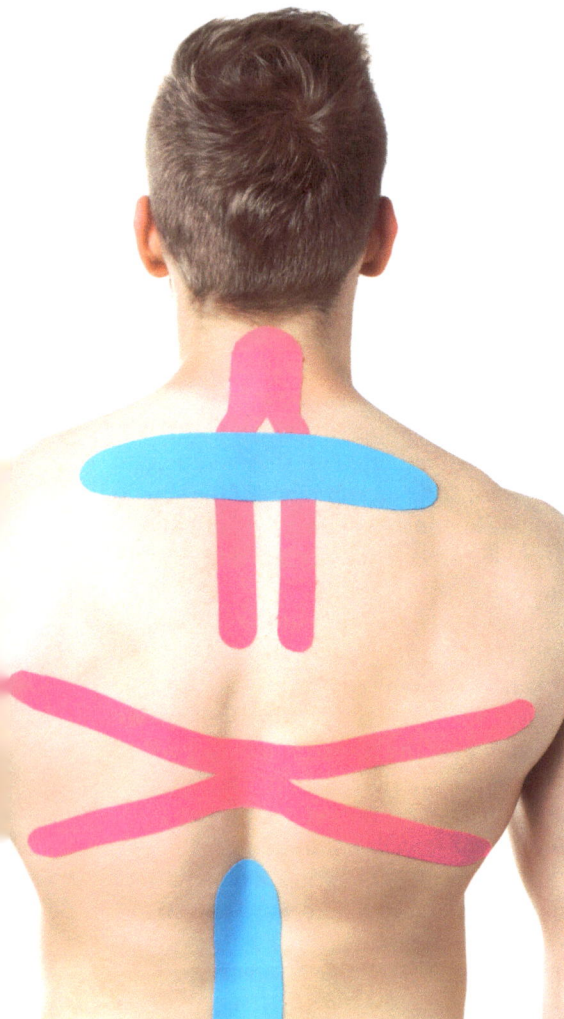

THE UTILIZATION OF FUNCTIONAL TAPE AND ITS EFFECT ON HUMAN PHYSIOLOGY

LYMPH

Functional Tape has been demonstrated effective for lymphatic drainage and edema reduction. This would be an application for acute patients who have experienced acute bruising, or for chronic edema patients who present with lymphedema associated with breast cancer for example. The physiologic mechanism by which the tape is effective for lymphatic drainage and the reduction of swelling is that the tape lifts the subdermal space of the skin allowing for drainage to occur. The tape assists in the removal of edema by directing exudates toward a lymph duct and by improving circulation and flow (Nakajima & Baldridge, 2013).

JOINTS

Taping provides immediate sensorimotor feedback regarding functional abilities. With the Functional Tape applied, patients often report symptom relief, improved comfort level, or stability of the involved joint. This sensory method supports joint physiology by exerting an effect on muscle function, enhancing endogenous analgesic mechanisms, as well as improving microcirculation (Slupik et al., 2007).

MUSCULATURE

Taping has been used to enhance muscle length in sites such as the ankle, knee, neck, shoulder girdle, upper limb and trunk. With the sensorimotor mechanism, the tape stimulates the mechanoreceptors in the skin and by reflex action, induces change in muscle tone (Mostert-Wentzel, 2012).

Gomez--Soriano (2013) demonstrated a short-term increase of EMG activity after treatment with Kinesio Tape, suggesting activation of central nervous system mechanisms, although without a therapeutic implication. The increased activity of the musculature, but not for therapeutic benefit, is a clinical rationale of why Functional Tape is effective in improving athletic performance.

Mostert-Wentzel (2012) also suggested that functional taping is a modality with the potential to improve athletic performance, when the sports activity depends on explosive muscle power. Maximum explosive power is the capability of the neuromuscular system to create a single maximum voluntary contraction at maximum speed. It is possible that cutaneous application of Functional Tape could improve muscle explosive power through increased sensory input to the neuromuscular system and increased activation of the sensorimotor reflex pathway.

PROPRIOCEPTION

Recent studies have documented significant effects on proprioception resulting from the application of Functional Tape (Chang et al., 2010). The term "proprioception" was first proposed by Sherrington in 1907(McCloskey, 1978). Proprioception described mechanoreceptors in the body that provide signal information relative to joint position and movement and also the perceived sensation of these forces by the central nervous system. Proprioception includes joint position sense, kinesthesia, and force sense. (Chang et al., 2010).

According to Chang et al. (2010) studies reveal that taping over the skin can stimulate cutaneous mechanoreceptors and deliver more signals to the central nervous system for information integration. The specialized receptors exist in skin, muscles, tendons, and joints. Proprioception can change with ageing, disease, injury, exercise training, and the use of external protective equipment or taping methods (Riemann & Lephart, 2002).

PAIN RESPONSE

Some studies report pain relief and therapeutic benefit with the use of Functional Tape, and others do not. The most frequently proposed hypothesis for pain reduction is the Gate Control Theory.

Functional taping generates a series of cutaneous afferents, which interfere with the transmission of mechanical and painful stimuli. This causes a differential stimulation of rapid nerve fibers, which activate a descending pain inhibitory pathway (Aguilar-Ferrandiz et al., 2014).

When a patient experiences "pain" they are having a subjective experience based upon their perception of noxious stimuli. Although the level of pain that the patient experiences is considered subjective, and will range in severity from patient to patient based upon their perception, objective physiologic changes are occurring at the site of pain, both with acute injuries and with patients who present with chronically injured tissues.

BIOMECHANICAL CHANGES ASSOCIATED WITH PAIN
(Sandstrom & Strachan, 2015)

1. The perception of pain is conveyed to the patient after an acute injury takes place or tissues are repetitively overloaded leading to a chronic pain presentation.
2. Inflammation and increased muscle contraction occurs at the site of injury.
3. Inhibition of proprioception of the injured tissue occurs.
4. Inhibited proprioception leads to poor muscle control at the site of "painful tissue."
5. With poor muscle control, poor articular biomechanics are noted.
6. Articular dysfunction leads to poor load application of the pain ful area.

With use of Functional Tape for patients who are experiencing pain, the tape can provide therapeutic benefit, which is great for the patient. And the application of Functional Tape can change the physiologic response to pain that the patient experiences.

The application of tape can lift the skin and decrease inflammation for acute injuries. It can also increase proprioception at the site of injured tissue for chronic patients.

By reducing edema and by increasing proprioception, the pathophysiologic response to pain that the patient experiences can be altered. This results in improved or normal function with optimized biomechanics.

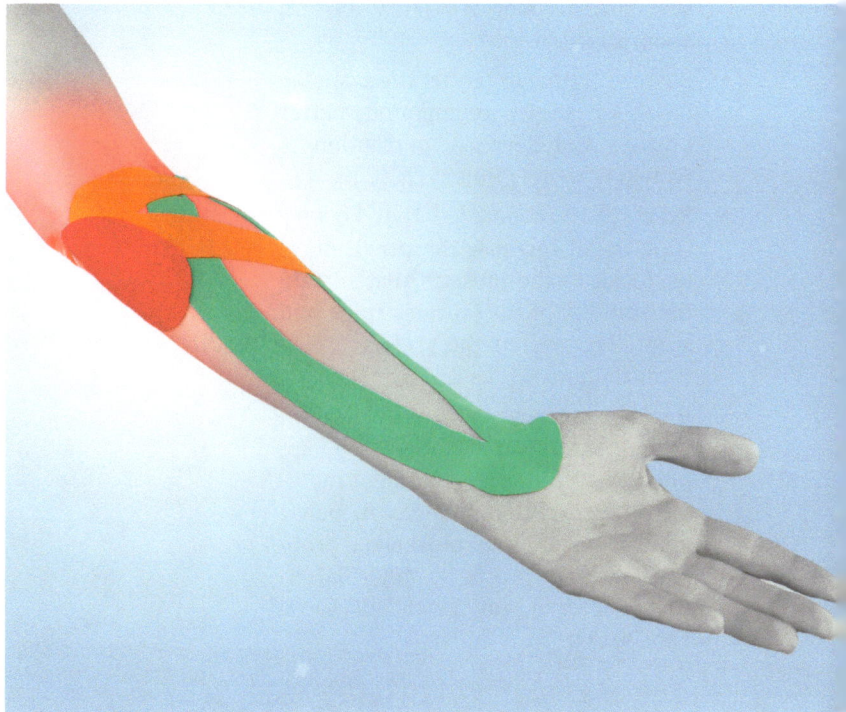

POSTURE TAPING FOR STRUCTURAL CORRECTION

Utilizing Functional Taping for structural correction, and to help patients create habits that support structural changes is the primary reason why we utilize Functional Tape at the American Posture Institute. Multiple different research studies have demonstrated that Functional Taping is an effective postural correction strategy, immediately effective in making postural changes with common postural distortion patterns.

Consider the following examples that have been demonstrated through research studies:

- The forward head posture angle has been shown to significantly decrease during computer work performed with neck retraction Posture Tape as compared to without Neck Retraction Tape (Yoo, 2013).

- Rounded shoulder Posture Taping with stretch has been shown to produce immediate mechanical correction of rounded shoulder posture in seated male workers (Han, Lee, & Yoon, 2015).

- Posture Taping to retract the scapulae has been shown to maintain better posture and decrease perception of pain in patients (Murray, 2005).

- Researchers concluded that Posture Tape might increase the provision of feedback to the muscles that sustain the stability of the thoracic spine and scapula as well as the preferred postural alignment (Lee & Yoo, 2011).

- It has been suggested that application of anterior pelvic tilt tape can be applied as an auxiliary treatment method for preventing changes in pelvic inclination and musculoskeletal problems of low back area by abnormal sitting posture in seated workers (Lee & Yoo, 2011).

Posture Taping, as explained by Clark (2014), is a part of the positioning system for paraplegic patients. It has proven very useful as a dynamic support, ideal during periods of growth or changes in functional status when existing equipment for compromised patients no longer adequately supports the patient. In these instances, Posture Taping can be an effective strategy to improve function, posture, positioning, and comfort of the patient (Clark, 2014).

Trotter (2013) explained that Functional Tape has a greater stimulatory effect with compromised tissue due to injury, fatigue, or poor posture. Applications of Posture Tape are used in cerebral palsy, brachial plexus palsy, and torticollis to facilitate normal postural alignment, to provide sensorial stimulation, to enhance functional motor skills, and to normalize muscle tone (Simsek et al., 2011).

One of the most important problems in cerebral palsied children is the disturbance of normal postural control mechanisms, which seriously affects their ability to perform functional activities and activities of daily living. Children with cerebral palsy often rely upon inappropriate control strategies and faulty feedback mechanisms when learning to maintain both static and dynamic sitting postures, which inevitably leads to postural distortion patterns, posture collapse, and functional dependency. Their posture systems cannot effectively control the body's position and motion in space because it lacks the ability to generate appropriate muscular force and to coordinate and integrate the sensory information received (Simsek et al., 2011). Posture Tape application for patients with cerebral palsy is used to enhance normal postural alignment by facilitating trunk stability, aiming to decrease their functional dependency.

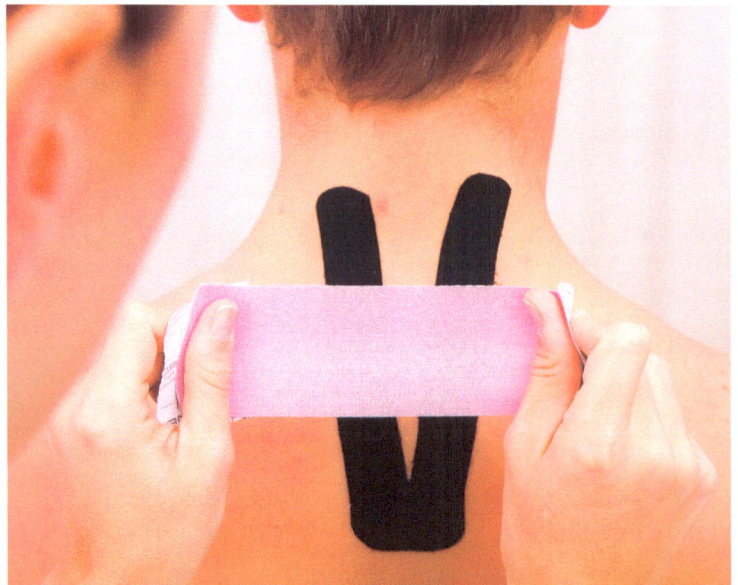

POSTURE TAPING OF THE POSTURE SYSTEM

The Posture System is the neuromusculoskeletal components of the human body responsible for holding the body upright against gravity. The Posture System is a complex and important system of the body allowing humans to resist gravity while static and during dynamic movements. The components work together in synchrony to balance the body against gravity while performing coordinates human movements.

The Posture System is divided into four posture quadrants, classified by their anatomic position. Each posture quadrant interacts with the quadrant above and below. Postural distortions of one posture quadrant frequently lead to compensatory postural distortion patterns of the other posture quadrants.

- **Posture Quadrant 1** is composed of the head and the cervical spine
- **Posture Quadrant 2** is composed of the upper extremities, the thoracic spine, and the thorax down to the diaphragm
- **Posture Quadrant 3** is composed of the lumbar spine, abdomen, and the pelvic girdle
- **Posture Quadrant 4** is composed of the lower extremities and feet

Now we will discuss a research review of the utilization of Functional Tape within each of the posture quadrants. We will discuss how Functional Tape does or does not affect the physiologic functions of each posture quadrant and relevant clinical considerations for your patients.

POSTURE QUADRANT 1

Primary anatomic markers of posture quadrant 1 that are relevant to Functional Taping include the cervical spine, the upper trapezius, and the sternocleidomastoid musculature. The primary physiologic function of posture quadrant 1 that is relevant to Functional Taping is to support the head upright against gravity in proper position over the shoulders.

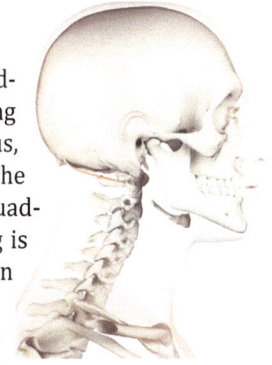

The primary postural distortion that occurs of the first posture quadrant is forward head posture, when the head is positioned anteriorly in relation to the shoulders. Other common postural distortions include lateral head flexion and head rotation. Physiologic compromise that occurs with forward head posture includes: tension headaches, suboccipital headaches, temporomandibular joint dysfunction, fatigue, muscular tension, neck pain, and cervical radiculopathy. Common consequences of head tilt include torticollis, neck pain, and muscular dysfunction.

Functional Taping that helps correct these posture distortions will be beneficial to the patient. The research indicates that the utilization of Functional Tape for postural correction and therapeutic benefit of posture quadrant 1 is beneficial. Let's review the literature first that supports the utilization for therapeutic benefit.

THERAPEUTIC BENEFITS OF POSTURE QUADRANT 1

It has been reported that the lifetime and point prevalence of neck pain are almost as high as those of low back pain. A systematic review of the literature has indicated that the 1-year prevalence of neck pain ranges between 16.7% and 75.1% with the mean average of 37.2% (Fejer et al., 2006). Additionally, mechanical neck pain results in substantial disability and costs in terms of medical costs and productivity lost (Saavedra-Hernandez, et al., 2012).

Saavedra-Hernandez et al. (2012) performed a research study evaluating the utilization of cervical spine manipulation and Kinesio tape for reduction of mechanical neck pain. Patients with mechanical neck pain who received cervical thrust manipulation or Kinesio Taping exhibited similar reductions in neck pain intensity and disability and similar changes in active cervical range of motion, except for rotation. Changes in neck pain surpassed the minimal clinically important difference, whereas changes in disability did not.

The results of this study suggest that the application of Kinesio Tape and cervical spine thrust manipulation had similar effects for reducing pain and disability. Additionally, patients in both groups experienced similar improvements in cervical flexion, extension, and lateral flexion in both directions. However, individuals who received the cervical thrust manipulation exhibited a greater increase in cervical rotation range of motion than those treated with Kinesio Tape. Nevertheless, changes in cervical range of motion were small, but the decrease in neck pain for both groups was statistically significant (Saavedra-Hernandez, et al., 2012).

The authors of the study suggest that the mechanism by which Kinesio Taping induced these changes is related to the neural feedback provided to the patients, which can facilitate their ability to move the cervical spine with a reduced mechanical irritation on the soft tissues. In addition, the tape might have created tension in soft tissue structures that provide afferent stimuli, facilitating a pain-inhibitory mechanism and thereby reducing the pain levels of the patients (Saavedra-Hernandez, et al., 2012).

According to Gonzalez-Iglesias et al. (2009), patients with acute whiplash associated disorders receiving an application of Kinesio Tape also exhibited statistically significant improvements in pain levels and cervical range of motion immediately following the application of Kinesio Tape and at a 24-hour follow-up. However, it is important to note that the improvements were small and may not be clinically meaningful to all patients suffering from whiplash.

This is a relevant consideration and therapeutic option if you see a lot of whiplash cases in your office. It has been reported that nearly 30% of whiplash patients continue to experience symptoms beyond 3 months, resulting in a considerable financial burden. Persistent pain and disability occur in up to 40% of patients who experience whiplash (Gonzalez-Iglesias et al., 2009).

Another study performed by Dawood et al. (2013) showed that the combined therapy of kinesio taping or cervical traction with exercise programs are effective in improving the absolute rotatory angle, pain intensity and function neck disability in mechanical neck dysfunction. This is an important consideration because both the utilization of tape with exercise and cervical traction with exercise is likely more effective for your patients than exercise recommendations alone.

It has been hypothesized that kinesio taping exerts its effects through increasing local circulation, reducing local edema, facilitating the targeted muscles, providing a positional stimulus to the skin, muscle, or fascial structures providing proper afferent input to the central nervous system. The findings of this study may be attributed to the effect of kinesio taping on proprioception as kinesio taping has an effect on cutaneous mechanoreceptors through stretching skin. This sense of stretching is thought to elaborate signal information for joint movement or joint position (Dawood et al., 2013).

STRUCTURAL AND FUNCTIONAL BENEFITS OF POSTURE QUADRANT 1

Now let's consider the utilization of Functional Tape for posture quadrant 1 and how it supports proper posture and/or contributes to the correction of postural distortion patterns.

The primary postural distortion of posture quadrant 1 is forward head posture. Yoo (2013) performed a research study demonstrating that the forward head posture angle significantly decreased during computer work performed with Neck Retraction Tape compared to without Neck Retraction Tape.

The upper trapezius muscle activity was also significantly decreased during computer work performed with Neck Retraction Tape compared to without. Yoo (2013) suggests that the taping tension provided by the Neck Retraction Tape may have provided a mechanical effect that prevented forward head posture while performing computer work. Neck Retraction Tape may also encourage a proper head posture in patients unfamiliar with the neck retraction posture contributing to posture habit re-education (Yoo, 2013).

This study showed that the upper trapezius muscle activity was also significantly decreased during computer work performed with Neck Retraction Tape compared to without. It is known that the blood and lymph circulations may be enhanced at the sites where Kinesio tape is applied; thus, the muscular and myofascial functions at those sites may also be affected.

The application of Kinesio tape to the skin may stimulate cutaneous mechanoreceptors, strengthen weakened muscles, and assist postural alignment. Neck Retraction Tape may stimulate cutaneous mechanoreceptors, causing forward head posture and a return to the standard head posture by enhancing the functions of the cervical extensor muscles that are commonly weak in patients who present with forward head posture. In addition, the tape likely provided a mechanical effect inhibiting forward head posture due the level of tension utilized (Yoo, 2013).

Ohman (2012) investigated the effects of Functional Taping in the correction of lateral head flexion associated with torticollis. The immediate reported effect of Kinesio taping was that it helped reduce the muscular imbalance of the lateral flexors of the cervical spine. He concluded that the tape has an immediate effect on muscular imbalance in infants with congenital muscular torticollis (Ohman, 2012).

POSTURE QUADRANT 2

Primary anatomic points of posture quadrant 2 that are relevant to Functional Taping include the shoulders, scapulae, and the upper extremities and the lower trapezius musculature. The primary physiologic functions of posture quadrant 2 that are relevant to Functional Taping are to stabilize the shoulder while freely moving the upper extremity, draw anteriorly rotated shoulders posteriorly, and lymphatic drainage with lymphedema.

The primary postural distortions that occur of the second posture quadrant are hyperkyphosis and anterior displacement of the shoulders associated with chest flexion. Other postural distortions that may occur include shoulder unleveling and abnormal lateral thoracic alignment.

Physiologic compromise that occurs due to postural distortion patterns of posture quadrant 2 included: asthma, decreased respiration, thoracic outlet syndrome, back pain, shoulder injuries, carpal tunnel syndrome, epicondylitis, muscular dysfunction, scoliosis, and the worst consequence associated with hyperkyphosis which is an increased rate of early mortality.

Functional Taping that helps correct these posture distortions and prevents these complications from occurring will be beneficial to the patient. The research indicates that the utilization of Functional Tape for postural correction and therapeutic benefit of posture quadrant 2 is beneficial. First, we will review the literature that supports the utilization for therapeutic benefit. There was minimal evidence for therapeutic benefit, but multiple studies showing benefit of the tape for structural and functional improvement.

THERAPEUTIC BENEFITS OF POSTURE QUADRANT 2

Lifetime prevalence of shoulder pain has been reported to range from 7% to 36% of the population. Rotator cuff pathology and subacromial impingement are among the most common diagnoses made in the shoulder region. The majority of cases are non-operative initially. Thelen et al. (2008) concluded that Functional Tape may be of some assistance to clinicians in improving pain-free active range of motion immediately after tape application for patients with shoulder pain. The utilization of Kinesio tape for decreasing pain intensity or disability for young patients with suspected shoulder tendonitis/impingement was NOT supported (Thelen et al., 2008).

Jaraczewska & Long (2006) demonstrated that the use of taping in conjunction with an established rehabilitation program may play an important role in the reduction of poststroke shoulder pain.

Kaya et al. (2011) suggest that Kinesio taping may be an alternative treatment option in the treatment of shoulder impingement syndrome especially when an immediate effect is needed. It was shown that Kinesio tape promotes the proximal stability of the scapula allowing free humeral movements without pain (Kaya et al., 2011).

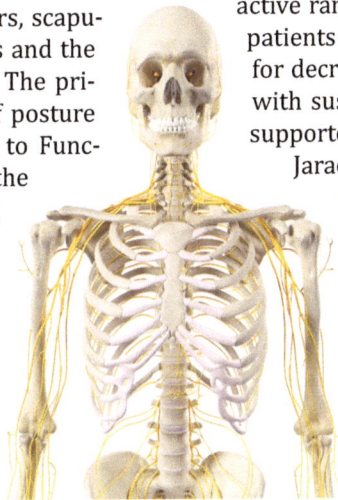

STRUCTURAL AND FUNCTIONAL BENEFITS OF POSTURE QUADRANT 2

The evidence is not overwhelmingly in favor of the utilization of Functional Tape for therapeutic benefit, but there are more studies showing structural and functional benefits that are also very important for the Posture Expert to consider.

Yasukawa et al. (2006) suggest that Kinesio tape is associated with improvement in upper extremity control and function in acute pediatric rehabilitation settings. The use of Kinesio tape as an adjunct to treatment may assist with goal-focused occupational therapy treatment during children's inpatient stay. The use of Kinesio taping in conjunction with the child's regular therapy program may favorably influence the cutaneous receptors of the sensorimotor system resulting in subsequent improvement of voluntary control and coordination of the upper limb (Yasukawa, Patel, & Sisung, 2006).

The application of Kinesio tape on the forearm appeared to enhance the force sense of forearm muscles immediately after application in healthy subjects. Although there was no statistically significant improvements in maximal grip, an enhanced force sense is of importance for competing athletes. Chang et al. (2010) suggest that Kinesio tape application may be used in competitive sports that require more precise hand force control such as pitching or shooting (Chang et al., 2010).

As explained before, Kaya et al. (2011) demonstrated that functional taping may be an alternative treatment option in the treatment of shoulder impingement syndrome especially when an immediate effect is needed. Shoulder impingement has been defined as compression and mechanical abrasion of the rotator cuff structures as they pass beneath the coracoacromial arch during elevation of the arm.

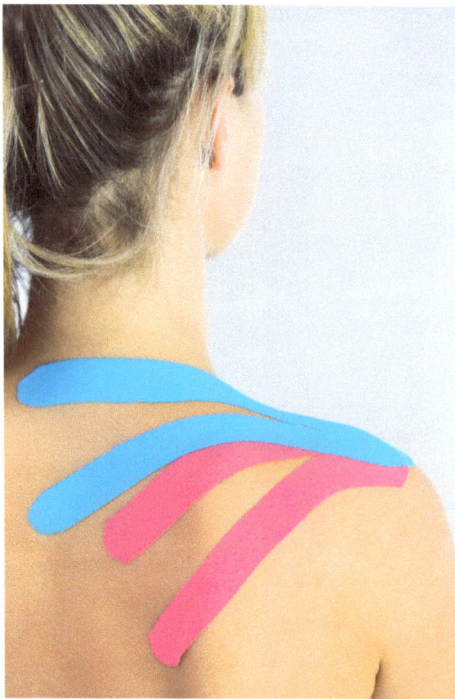

Multiple theories have been proposed to explain the primary etiology of shoulder impingement, including anatomic abnormalities of the coracoacromial arch or humeral head, "tension overload," ischemia, or degeneration of the rotator cuff tendons; and shoulder kinematic abnormalities. Inflammation in the suprahumeral space, inhibition of the rotator cuff muscles, damage to the rotator cuff tendons, and altered kinematics are believed to exacerbate the condition. Kinematic changes have been thought to be present in patients with impingement syndrome and to result in narrowing of the supraspinatus muscle outlet or suprahumeral space.

One of the aims of Functional Tape in this case is to normalize the scapulohumeral rhythm by altering the scapular muscle activity and correcting abnormal scapular position. The activity of the lower trapezius was found to be increased in baseball players with shoulder impingement syndrome. It has been proposed that the control of scapula and the shoulder could be provided by the constant proprioceptive feedback and alignment correction during dynamic movements with Kinesio taping. It has been shown that Kinesio tape promotes the proximal stability of the scapula allowing free humeral movements without pain. (Kaya et al., 2011).

Jaraczewska & Long (2006) conclude that the use of Functional Taping protocols in conjunction with an established rehabilitation program may play an important role in the reduction of poststroke shoulder pain, soft tissue inflammation, muscle weakness, and postural malalignment. The authors of this study believe that the tape may improve the position of the glenohumeral joint and may provide the proprioceptive feedback to achieve proper body alignment. These factors are fundamental when exercises to restore the upper extremity functions are performed (Jaraczewska & Long, 2006).

Patients diagnosed with stroke often present with a combination of muscle weakness or muscle imbalance, decreased postural control, muscle spasticity, poor voluntary control, and body misalignment. The ability of the adult with stroke to functionally use the affected arm may be diminished due to all of the above problems. As clinicians, we need to be aware that regaining functional use of the upper extremity after a stroke is one of the most challenging tasks for the patient and for the therapist working with the patient. For the upper extremity to perform its functional tasks, the trunk needs to be held upright and needs to be able to move freely from one stable position to another either against the pull of the gravity or despite its pull.

Two groups of muscles are responsible for trunk control. There are back extensors posteriorly and abdominal muscle anteriorly. When the upper extremity performs its functional activity, it requires efficient function of the abdominal muscles to maintain and achieve a desired movement. For the abdominal muscles to act efficiently, they need a stable thorax. With increased thoracic kyphosis, the insertion and origin of the obliques is approximated, therefore the muscles cannot function in full capacity.

It is important to mention that an excessive kyphotic position of the thoracic spine caused by poor posture, muscle weakness, or muscle imbalance will cause a compression of the rib cage. Such compression will reduce the volume of the lungs and cause the patient to fatigue easily. When evaluating the upper extremity function, one has to include postural assessment. Alignment of the cervical, thoracic, and lumbar spine influences scapular position and the overall upper extremity function (Jaraczewska & Long, 2006).

The Kinesio taping method in conjunction with other therapeutic interventions may facilitate or inhibit muscle function, support joint structure, reduce pain, and provide proprioceptive feedback to achieve and maintain preferred body alignment. Restoring trunk and scapula alignment after the stroke is critical in an effective treatment program for the upper extremity in hemiplegia (Jaraczewska & Long, 2006).

Hsu et al. (2009) noted positive effects on both scapular muscle activity and motion performance after the application of Kinesio taping. The results suggest that scapular tape affects the muscle activity of the upper trapezius, anterior deltoid, and serratus anterior, and that the effects are related to proprioception feedback. These results implicate that the mechanisms by which scapular taping induces effects can be explained by neuromuscular control and proprioceptive feedback factors.

Lin et al. (2011) suggest that the rationale for taping is that it affords protection and support for a joint during functional movement. Although it is unclear if tape protects the glenohumeral joint position, immediate symptoms improve with scapular taping and relief of symptoms is greater during functional movement than in static positions. These results showed significant changes in EMG activity in the scapular muscles with the application of tape in the asymptomatic group. Propri-

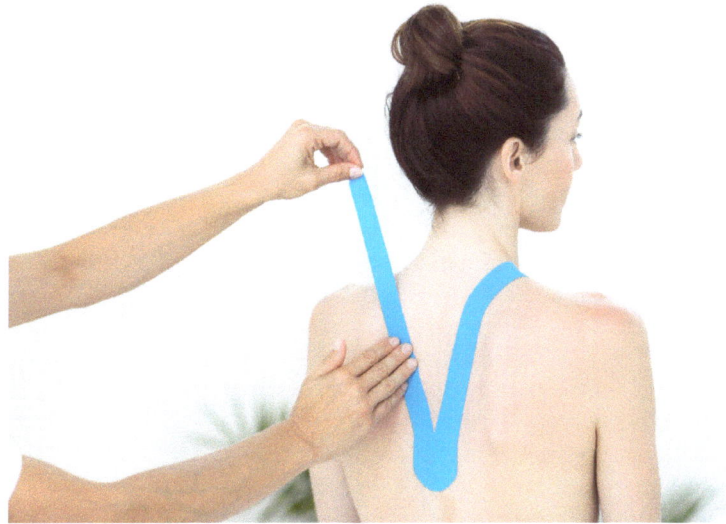

oceptive feedback was also enhanced with taping. Thus, the mechanisms by which scapular taping can be explained are neuromuscular control as well as proprioceptive feedback factors (Lin et al., 2011).

With further consideration of scapular stabilization, Cote et al. (2013) have shown that wearing a scapular brace improved shoulder posture and scapular muscle activity, but EMG changes were highly variable. It was concluded that the use of a scapular brace or tape in a cross formation might improve shoulder posture and muscle activity in overhead athletes with poor posture (Cole et al., 2013).

A similar study showed that when Functional Tape was applied to the scapulae of competitive female handball players, positive changes in scapular motion were noted. This was a suggested therapy to prevent shoulder injuries. The tape had a large effect on posterior tilting and upward rotation of the scapulae. The scapula is the most important link between the upper extremity and the axial skeleton. Abnormal movement of the scapula can predispose overhead athletes to shoulder injuries (Van Herzeele, 2013).

The purpose of this exam performed by Han et al. (2015) was to examine the changes in pectoralis minor length, the supine measurement of rounded shoulder posture, and the total scapular distance in seated male workers with rounded shoulder posture, after rounded-shoulder-taping using kinesiology tape with stretch for the experimental group and without stretch for placebo taping.

Kinesio taping with stretch significantly increased the pectoralis minor length and significantly decreased the supine measurement of rounded shoulder posture and total scapular distance; taping without stretch did not. Using Kinesio tape with stretch produces immediate postural correction of rounded shoulder posture in seated male workers (Han, Lee, & Yoon, 2015).

THE UTILIZATION OF FUNCTIONAL TAPE FOR LYMPH DRAINAGE

The utilization of Functional Tape for lymph drainage is of particular importance in posture quadrant 2. Some papers demonstrate the effectiveness of Functional Tape for this purpose, and others do not. The research is not conclusive; be sure to consider this application from both points of view.

25% of breast cancer patients suffer from the complication of lymphedema. Lymphedema is defined as arm edema in the breast cancer patient caused by interruption of the flow of the axillary lymphatic system from surgery or radiation therapy, which results in the accumulation of fluid in the subcutaneous tissue of the arm, with a decrease in tissue distensibility around the joints and an increased weight of the extremity (Taradaj, 2014).

Taradaj (2014) explains that the utilization of Kinesio tape had a significant effect on the reduction of lymphedema and accelerated healing effects compared to standard methods.

Another study suggests that Functional Tape could replace the bandage used in decongestive lymphatic therapy, and it could be an alternative choice for the breast-cancer-related lymphedema patient with poor short-stretch bandage compliance.

sai et al. (2009) explain that more efficient treatment protocols are needed for clinical practice. The usage of Kinesio tape was better than the bandage, and benefits included longer wearing time, less difficulty in usage, and increased comfort and convenience (Tsai et al., 2009).

On the contrary, Smykla (2013) concluded that the edema reduction of multilayered bandages was much better than in results observed in taping groups. The Kinesio tape appeared to be ineffective at secondary lymphedema after breast cancer treatment in this study. The single-blind, controlled pilot study results suggested that Kinesio tape could not replace the bandage, and at this moment it should not be an alternative choice for the breast cancer-related lymphedema patient (Smykla, 2013).

POSTURE QUADRANT 3

Primary anatomic markers of posture quadrant 3 that are relevant to Functional Taping include the lumbar spine, the pelvis, and the lumbar erector spinae and oblique musculature. The primary physiologic function of posture quadrant 3 that is relevant to Functional Taping is to support the trunk and pelvis upright against gravity in a position that allows for efficient ambulation of the lower extremity.

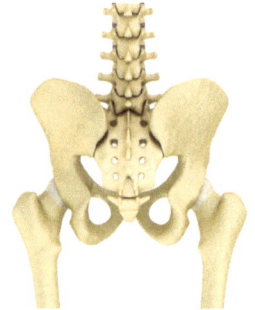

The primary postural distortions that occur of the third posture quadrant are anterior and posterior pelvic tilt associated with an increase or decrease of the lumbar lordosis. Another common postural distortions is pelvic unleveling in which one side of the pelvis appears to be higher than the other.

Physiologic compromise that occurs with posture distortions of posture quadrant 3 include: back pain, lumbar radiculopathy, sciatica, scoliosis, digestive issues, increased menstrual pain, urinary incontinence, and lumbar and pelvic muscular dysfunction patterns.

Functional Taping that helps correct these posture distortions will be beneficial to the patient in addition to their complete postural correction protocol. The research indicates that the utilization of Functional Tape for postural correction and therapeutic benefit of this posture quadrant is beneficial. Let's review the literature first that supports the utilization for therapeutic benefit.

THERAPEUTIC BENEFITS OF POSTURE QUADRANT 3

Low back pain is a very significant musculoskeletal condition affecting millions of people. The burden of costs associated with low back pain is at a record high worldwide.

Functional Taping has been shown to reduce disability and pain in people with chronic non-specific low back pain. At one week, the experimental group that utilized the tape had significantly greater improvement in disability on the Oswestry score and on the Roland-Morris score. Similarly trunk muscle endurance was significantly better at one week after the tape application (Castro-Sanchez et al., 2012).

Posture Experts should be aware that although immediate therapeutic benefits were noted, these effects were not significant four weeks later.

STRUCTURAL AND FUNCTIONAL BENEFITS OF POSTURE QUADRANT 3

The structural and functional benefits of utilizing posture tape for posture quadrant 3 will be of high clinical value to Posture Experts. The correction of pelvic and lumbar postural distortion patterns is of utmost importance for the maintenance of long-term postural correction of your patients.

Lee and Yoo (2011) suggest that application of anterior pelvic tilt tape to assist in correcting posterior pelvic tilt can be applied as an auxiliary treatment method for preventing changes in pelvic inclination and musculoskeletal problems of low back area associated with awkward sitting posture in seated workers (Lee & Yoo, 2011).

Posterior pelvic tilt specifically reduces lordosis by flexing the lumbar spine, which causes posterior movement of the nucleus pulposus and an increase in the intervertebral foramina diameter. When lumbar lordosis is decreased, imbalance in the center of gravity of the anterior to the sacrum may be created (Lee et al., 2011).

This is relevant because prolonged sitting decreases the lumbar lordotic curve and increases intradiscal pressure, pressure on the ischium, and muscle activity. It has been reported that prolonged flexion during sitting was the cause of redistribution of the nucleus within the annulus. Such factors together may eventually cause disc herniation, degeneration, or rupture that commonly lead to low back pain. Moreover, a prolonged static sitting posture may have a negative effect on the nutrition of the intervertebral disc.

The erector spinae and the internal oblique muscles to which the tape was applied in this study are the muscles that stabilize sacroiliac joint. The erector spinae may increase lumbar lordosis by causing anterior tilt of the pelvis, since it is attached to the sacrum and pelvis. The upper anterior fibers of the internal obliques, which are fixed at the thorax, may also contribute to anterior pelvic tilt.

It is known that the blood and lymph circulations may be enhanced at the sites where the tape is applied, and thus the muscular and myofascial functions at those sites may be affected. The application of functional tape to the skin may stimulate cutaneous mechanoreceptors, strengthen the weakened muscles, and assist postural alignment. Thus, even in postures such as slumped sitting, where external resistance causes posterior pelvic tilt, Posture Tape may stimulate cutaneous mechanoreceptors, causing anterior pelvic tilt by enhancing the functions of the external obliques and internal oblique muscles (Lee & Yoo, 2011).

Most seated workers adopt the relaxed or slumped sitting posture during long hours of deskwork. Clinically, it is known that passive postures such as slump sitting aggravate chronic low back pain. Posture Tape has been shown to increase the feedback to the muscles that sustain the stability of the thoracic spine and scapula as well as the preferred postural alignment to prevent low back pain. For both male and female participants, anterior pelvic tilt taping increased the anterior inclination of the pelvis on both sides (Lee et al., 2011).

Other studies conducted, demonstrate an increase in muscle activity, improved range of motion, and better flexibility with the application of Posture Tape. Lemos et al. (2014) demonstrated that Kinesio tape influenced fascia mobility, allowing for slight improvement of lumbar flexibility.

Paoloni and colleagues (2011) also found that the application of tape over trunk extensor muscles could help restore normal levels of extensor muscle activation in full trunk flexion in patients with low back pain.

Yoshida and Kahanov (2007) suggest that Functional Tape may increase active range of motion of lower trunk flexion. The specific Y taping technique with attachment at the sacrum followed by stretching of the tape in extension used in this study may be beneficial in increasing the flexibility of trunk flexion. Additional taping techniques such as a Y or straight technique placed while the participant is in extension or lateral flexion should be investigated to ascertain whether these techniques are more appropriate for those motions (Yoshida & Kahanov, 2007).

Finally, Cepeda et al. reported that the application of Functional Tape to abdominal muscles in children with hypotonia is a therapeutic approach facilitating the transition from supine position to sitting. Allowing them to perform their activities of daily living more efficiently.

POSTURE QUADRANT 4

Primary anatomic markers of posture quadrant 4 that are relevant to Functional Taping include the quadriceps, hamstings, knee, and calcaneus. The primary physiologic function of posture quadrant 4 that is relevant to Functional Taping is to support the body upright against gravity while static, and to perform accurate cycles of gait so the patient has coordinated ambulatory movements.

The primary postural distortion that occurs of the fourth posture quadrant is pronation of the feet bilaterally, or one individual foot. It is important to note that a common observation of postural asymmetry is when patients present with a short leg. This presentation, however, is much more commonly associated with pelvic unleveling of posture quadrant 3 than anatomic discrepancies of posture quadrant 4.

Physiologic compromise that occurs with posture distortions of posture quadrant 4 includes: recurrent ankle sprains, knee osteoarthritis, plantar fasciitis, uncoordinated gait patterns, and muscular tension of the major muscle groups of the lower extremity.

Functional Taping that helps correct posture distortions, improving function of the lower extremity, will be beneficial to the patient in addition to their complete postural correction protocol. The research indicates that the utilization of Functional Tape for postural correction and therapeutic benefit of this posture quadrant is beneficial in many cases. Let's review the literature first that supports the utilization for therapeutic benefit.

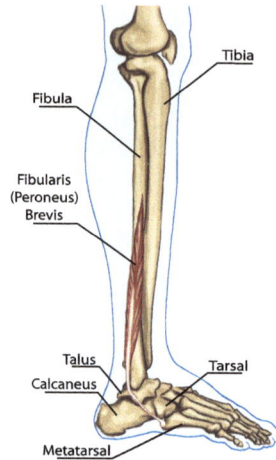

THERAPEUTIC BENEFITS OF POSTURE QUADRANT 4

Of the literature review that was conducted, evidence of therapeutic relief for posture quadrant 4 was limited to the knee. The therapeutic effects of knee taping included minimization of pain, increased muscle strength, improved gait pattern and enhanced functional outcome of patients with sports injury, osteoarthritis, and patellofemoral pain (Tieh-Cheng, Fu et al., 2008).

Structural and Functional Benefits of Posture Quadrant 4

Functional correction has been shown in the literature for posture quadrant 4. However, structural correction of the primary postural distortion of posture quadrant 4, pronation, was not shown to be improved with the application of Functional Tape. According to Luque-Suarez (2014), Kinesio taping does not correct foot pronation compared with sham kinesio taping protocols in people with pronated feet.

Let's consider the utilization of Functional Tape on the ankle.

Sports injuries comprise 8% of pediatric emergency department visits and 41% of emergency department visits for musculoskeletal complaints are sports related Injuries to the ankle are the most common sports related injury, making up 20% of injuries induced by sports-related activity. These injuries to the ankle include sprains, at 34% of ankle injuries, contusions at 30%, and fractures at 25% (Elshemy & Bettecha, 2013).

Ankle sprains usually happen when there is a sudden movement or twist, and often when the foot rolls over. A sudden movement or twist can overstretch the ligaments, causing tears, bruising, and swelling around the joint. These movements are more likely to happen when a person is running, jumping or quickly changing direction in sports such as basketball and football. Sports involving contact and jumping have the highest injury levels.

A previous study found that after an ankle sprain, up to 40% of sufferers continue to report residual disability which might persist for seven years after the original inversion trauma (Elshemy & Bettecha, 2013). Functional ankle instability involves mechanical, muscular, and sensorimotor deficiencies. Peroneal muscle weakness was the most significant factor contributing to recurrent ankle sprains.

Peroneal strengthening has been advocated for many years in the rehabilitation of both acute and chronic ankle sprains. The high incidence of lateral ankle sprains and the high rate of reinjury have prompted many researchers to examine the possible causes for this chronic instability. Three causes of instability have been suggested: a decrease in muscular strength of the ankle everters, an increase in lateral ligamentous laxity, and proprioceptive deficits resulting from a disruption in the integrity of the joint mechanoreceptors.

Decline in dynamic position sense is associated with decrease in the balance and this decline in proprioception can be prevented or improved by proprioceptive training. Proprioception based rehabilitation programs could improve functional status causing independent changes in the joint. A study was conducted by Elshemy and Bettecha (2013) that compared the effect of Kinesio tape versus proprioceptive training of the ankle on pediatric patients that present with functional ankle instability.

The post-treatment results of the study group A reinforced the effectiveness of Kinesio Taping on improving dynamic position sense of the ankle in children with functional ankle instability. The application of Kinesio tape can be used to produce increased sensory stimulation of the mechanoceptors in ligaments and tendons to assist motion while relying on the stretched tape for corrective posture.

This concept underlies the hypotheses that proprioception will be enhanced through increased cutaneous feedback from the Kinesio tape, thus facilitating the subject's ability to more accurately reposition themselves to the previous target position. The improvement seen in the study group A, thus may be due to the effect of taping on providing immediate sensorimotor feedback through direct contact between the skin and tape. Its elastic properties may cause proprioceptive stimulation anticipating a facilitory effect of cutaneous mechanoreceptors. Some research suggests Kinesio tape as a useful therapeutic and prophylactic assistance in rehabilitation and during activity (Elshemy & Bettecha, 2013).

Briem et al (2011) found similar results, that Functional Tape may enhance dynamic muscle support of the ankle. The efficacy of Kinesio tape in preventing an-

kle sprains via the same mechanism, however, was found to be unlikely, as the tape had no effect on muscle activation of the fibularis longus (Briem et al., 2011).

Tests of postural control have shown that individuals with ankle instability have poorer frontal plane stability than those with unaffected ankles. Due to their role as the primary everters and dynamic stabilizers of the ankle, the function of the fibularis (peroneus) muscles in relation to ankle stability and lateral sprains has been extensively studied.

The mechanism responsible for improving postural control with the application of tape or bracing may be stimulation of the cutaneous exteroreceptors from the foot and ankle. It has also been proposed that greater preactivation of the fibularis muscles prior to inversion stress may overcome the electromechanical delay, which could result in a larger spindle response. Nonelastic adhesive tape has been used for injury prevention and during rehabilitation after ankle injury (Briem et al., 2011).

Fayson et al. (2012) concluded that the application of Kinesio tape to the ankle may improve static restraint in the ankle joint without altering peak motion or dynamic postural control.

On the contrary, another study observed no relevant changes following application of Kinesio tape to the ankle. There was a minimal demonstration of improved postural control following tape application, but enough for Shields et al. (2013) to recommend the use of Kinesio Tape to treat balance deficits associated with ankle instability.

Huang et al (2011) observed differences when applying Kinesio and placebo tape to the ankle. The results showed that vertical ground reaction force and EMG activity of medial gastrocnemius significantly increased during the jumping task when Kinesio tape

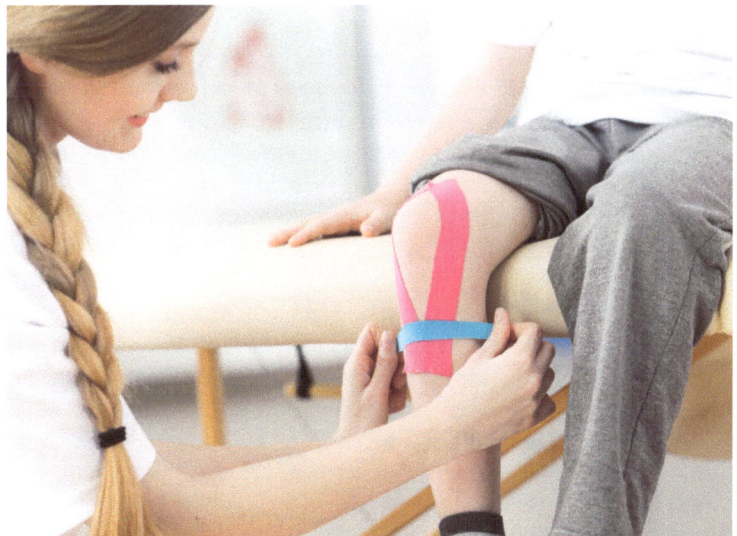

was applied. The placebo taping caused a significant decrease in jump height and no change in EMG activity of all testing muscles and vertical ground reaction force. Different types of elastic tape caused varied effects during exercise activity. The distinct structure and degree of elasticity would produce different biomechanical effects.

Nakajima and Baldridge (2013) found different results. They found that Functional tape application on the ankle neither decreased nor increased vertical jump height in healthy non-injured young individuals, but did increase dynamic postural control in females for certain directions.

In this current study, the main difference between the control and experimental group was the existence of tension in the Functional Tape for the experimental group compared to the lack of tension in the control group. It is a possibility that the tension provided by the real application might have increased the neural feedback to the participants during ankle movement, facilitating increased balance. Tactile input has been shown to alter motor control by changing the excitability of the central nervous system. This is in accordance with the claim that the tape applied with tension in the direction of the muscle fibers would facilitate the strength of the underlying muscles (Nakajima & Baldridge, 2013).

Multiple studies have been produced showing the effects, or non-effects of the utilization of Posture Tape on the ankle. Now consider the utilization of tape on the larger muscular groups of the lower extremity.

In a preliminary study, it was found that Kinesio tape applied to the anterior aspect of the thigh could significantly enhance the joint active range of motion and that this increase is correlated with an increase in surface EMG of the muscles of the anterior compartment of the thigh, the quadriceps femoris muscle (Kase, 1994).

Another researcher found, however, that Kinesio taping on the anterior thigh neither decreased nor increased muscle strength in healthy non-injured young athletes (Tieh-Cheng Fu et al., 2008).

It was also shown that Kinesio tape applied to the gluteus maximus muscle of healthy young male athletes significantly increases short-term vertical jump height for explosive muscle power over time. Kinesio tape improves short-term muscle power of the gluteus maximus directly after application and 30 minutes later. Although the improvements in jump height may appear small, even differences of this magnitude can influence athletes at high-performance levels.

The main effect of Kinesio tape in this case is attributed to applying the tape with tension. This provides a pulling force, which causes a change in stretch load, pressure and shear force, triggering the mechanoreceptors in the subdermal soft tissue and fascia. The central nervous system integrates the sensory input, and modulates gamma-motor firing, which in turn leads to increased muscle tone (Mostert-Wentzel, 2012).

VENOUS INSUFFICIENCY

Another common use for the utilization of Functional Tape in posture quadrant 4 is for venous symptoms of the lower extremity. This can be very painful and debilitating for your patients, finding a non-invasive approach to care for these patients is within good practice guidelines.

Venous insufficiency is characterized by persistent lower limb venous hypertension as a consequence of venous reflux and/or obstruction, a calf muscle pump function failure and ankle motion restriction. Prolonged venous hypertension can increase calf muscle impairment and produce pain, perception of heaviness, nocturnal cramps, "restless leg" syndrome, pruritus pain, and edema.

17% of elderly pateitns present with venous insufficiency. Given the elevated incidence of chronic venous insufficiency there is an urgent need to establish effective prevention and treatment protocols to meet the growing demand for care of these patients (Aguilar--Ferrandiz et al., 2014).

A research study was conducted in which the experimental group received Kinesio taping. Patients were in prone position and the tape direction was from origin to insertion at tensions ranging from 15% to 50% (Aguilar-Ferrandiz et al., 2014). At four weeks after application of a mixed Kinesio taping-compression model, chronic venous insufficiency patients showed a significantly reduced degree of reflux and edema and a significant improvement in venous symptoms, pain intensity, severity, physical function and body pain in comparison to pretreatment values and to the outcomes of a placebo Kinesio taping application. The author concluded that application of the ta[e three times per week reduces venous specific symptoms, pain and severity (Aguilar-Ferrandiz et al., 2014).

CLINICAL ANALYSIS FOR THE UTILIZATION OF POSTURE TAPE

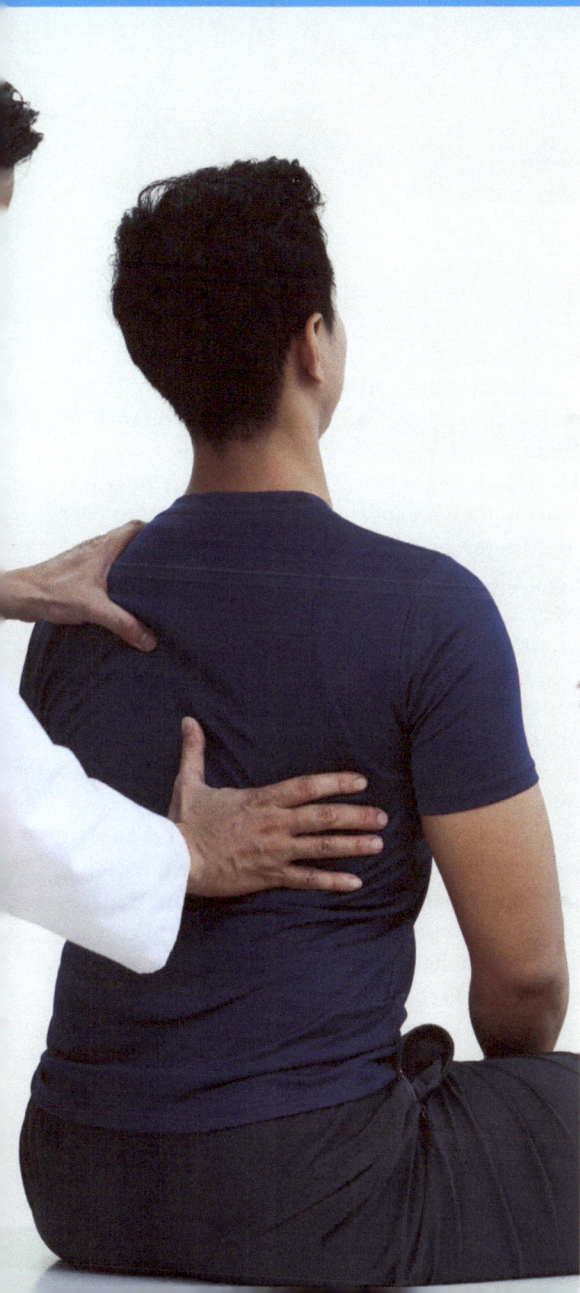

At this point we have discussed why you would consider using Functional Tape with your patients, and how it works. We have discussed the theories explaining why Functional Tape is effective for different case presentations, ranging from lymphedema to increased gluteus muscle contraction. We have looked at the Posture System and reviewed what literature supports the utilization of tape for different case presentations within each of the posture quadrants.

As we begin Module 3, and continue on into Module 4, the information presented will be highly applicable for clinical practice. The information that you can take and use right away with your patients. We will discuss how to analyze which of your patients need what kind of tape and at what tension it should be applied. In Module 3 we will also review the different types of tape that are available on the market and the features of these different tapes so you can make an educated decision of what tape to have in your office.

Many Posture Experts wonder how the same tape can have so many different functions. Put simply, the tension of the tape makes all the difference. The tape can be applied from 0% tension up to 80% tension, depending upon the clinical objective that you hope to achieve with your patient. In this module we will discuss the different tape tensions and how they are relevant to the application of Functional Tape.

Then in Module 4 we will discuss how to apply the tape for many different conditions of the posture system. We will demonstrate therapeutic applications for common, chronic pain conditions as well as Posture Taping protocols for the most common postural distortion patterns that patients present with. In many cases we will show multiple methods, you can pick and choose what taping protocols you prefer to use in your office.

When beginning to utilize Functional tape in your practice, determine what your clinical objective is first. At the American Posture Institute we primarily utilize taping for purposes of posture habit re-education. Meaning that the tape is a tool to help remind the patient to maintain proper posture during their daily activities. It is a kinesthetic tool in which the patient actually feels better posture, prompting them to maintain proper postural design during their normal activities.

We also utilize Posture Tape with our patients in the dynamic phase of their postural correction treatment plan to help the patient maintain proper posture while performing functional movements. Because the tape is functional, it won't restrict the patient while they are performing their postural rehabilitation exercises.

Posture tape is utilized in this case to improve performance and assist in retraining dynamic postural patterns.

Posture taping, when used in this manner is not therapeutic. The clear objective is to improve postural distortions of the posture quadrant in which the tape is applied. Every once in awhile however, at the American Posture Institute we will utilize tape for therapeutic purposes when deemed appropriate with certain patients. Tape is utilized for therapeutic purposes if the patient meets one the following criteria: they present with chronic localized pain that has not regressed with treatment or to assist in controlling swelling and lymphatic drainage.

It is important to note that there are therapeutic affects of the application of Functional Tape, many of which we covered in module 2. This is a viable option for patient management that should not be discounted. Especially for your chronic

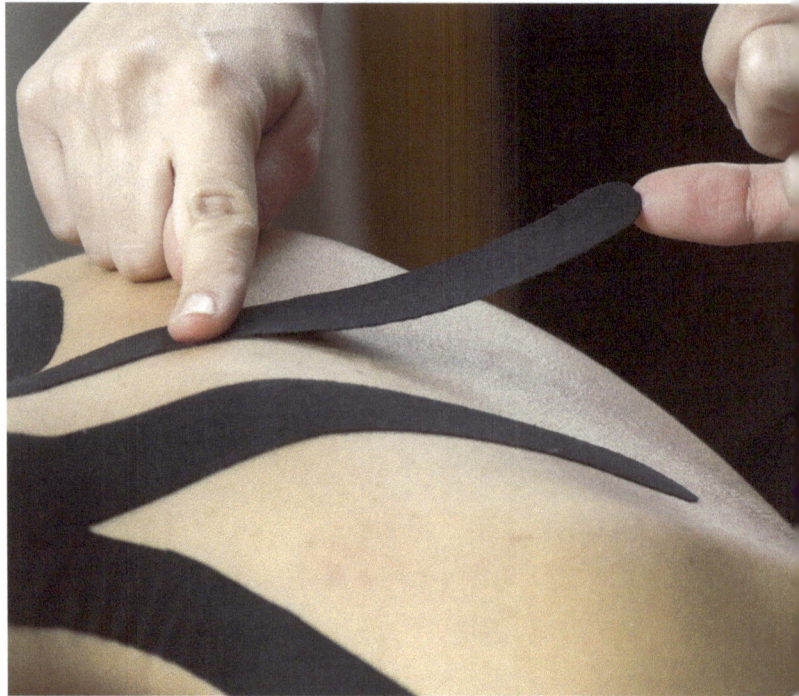

patients who have not had the subjective changes in pain that they desire.

Fixing pain is not our first priority at the American Posture Institute, however for many patients getting out of pain is their top priority. We focus on objective correction of the postural distortion patterns that they present with on their baseline posture images. With the far majority of patients, when you correct their postural distortion patterns they will also experience pain relief. With certain patients this is not the case. After performing these patients' re-evaluations we make the clinical decision to use tape for therapeutic relief if necessary.

You, the Posture Expert must be clear in your treatment decisions and what the expected outcome is. Decide where you want to focus your attention and the most efficient ways to get your patients back to a healthy state. How you want to serve the patients in your office is your choice, which is exciting, the opportunities are endless and should be a reflection of you. There is no one way, or panacea. Postural correction is not a one size fits all model, it changes everyday based upon the presentation of your patients and the skills and knowledge that you acquire as a Posture Expert.

When utilizing tape for the specific purpose of postural correction you then need to decide what postural distortion pattern you want to focus on correcting. It is recommended to wait until the patient has had a re-evaluation before utilizing Functional Tape. Their primary postural distortion patterns may change after they begin a treatment plan of complete posture correction. We will discuss treatment plans in much more detail in Module 4.

At the re-evaluation during the Structural Restoration phase of postural correction care, determine what postural distortion pattern is the most prominent based on the information collected from their posture images and visual posture analyses. Compare the images on the re-evaluation to their baseline images of their initial visit. Which postural distortions demonstrate less objective correction and would benefit the most from the application of the tape?

Also consider your patients' occupational activities and how they can benefit the greatest from the utilization of the tape in terms of posture habit re-education. For example, if your patient is a desk worker and presents with forward head posture, the utilization of neck retraction Posture Tape would be a good option for objective correction and for posture habit re-education. For patients who are training for certain sports, such as runners, they would likely benefit from Proprioceptive Functional Taping protocols of posture quadrants 3 and 4. These taping decisions are congruent with what the patient does each day, and the results they are working to obtain.

Once your patient has advanced to the dynamic phase of postural correction care, re-test how they perform functional human movements on the re-evaluation. If they present with a significant postural collapse during a particular movement, you can utilize the tape to stimulate the area of postural collapse and draw the patient's conscious and subconscious awareness to this area for performance enhancement purposes.

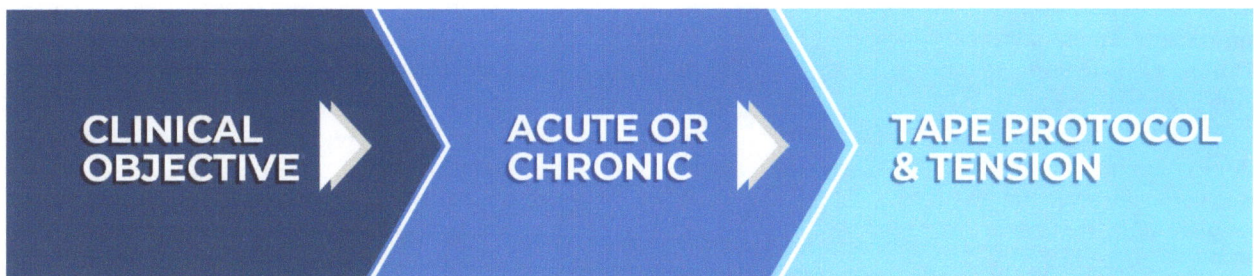

3 STEP ANALYSIS

There are endless application opportunities for the utilization of Functional Tape. Again, be clear on your clinical objectives with each patient that you utilize the tape for. Once you have determined that clinical objective, then you must classify the patient as acute or chronic, and determine what tension of the tape to utilize.

STEP 1: DEFINE THE CLINICAL OBJECTIVE

You have been working with the patient, you know what postural distortions they still present with, and what symptoms they are or are not experiencing. Will it benefit the patient the most to utilize tape for postural correction, performance enhancement, or therapeutic relief. Keep in mind, these three categories are assuming that the patient is not an acute, hypermobile patient. In this case it is recommended to use restrictive, traditional tape to prevent further injury.

The clinical objective of postural correction is to improve their primary postural distortion pattern and to re-educate their habits causing postural collapse during their daily activities. Research demonstrates that Functional Tape is effective in structural correction, and we know from experience that when a patient can FEEL better posture, they are prompted to maintain this correct position.

Do you have patients who fall into this category?

The second group is proprioceptive enhancement. These patients are often athletes, but are certainly not limited to athletes. This group of patients demonstrates dysfunction during range of motion or muscle testing, or demonstrates palpable muscular dysfunction. This type of taping is also used frequently during the dynamic postural correction phase in which the patient is working to improve their posture during motion. Performance based objectives are utilized to monitor the patient's progress.

The third group is therapeutic. The clinical objective for this group is to relieve pain. Patients in this group are the type of patients who have chronic, recurrent pain despite objective improvement of postural correction. Meaning, they show objective results, but their subjective pain levels are still high.

CLINICAL OBJECTIVE ▶ **ACUTE OR CHRONIC** ▶ **TAPE PROTOCOL & TENSION**

STEP 2: DETERMINE ACUTE OR CHRONIC

Consider the patient's case presentation and determine if they are in acute or chronic pain or acute or chronic biomechanical dysfunction. Acute patients have different clinical objectives and should be clinically treated differently than a chronic patient.

If the patient is acute, determine whether they need Restrictive Tape or Functional Tape first. If they are hypermobile they fall within the category of Restrictive Tape. If the goal is to reduce muscle spasmodic activity or to reduce swelling, then functional tape would be used.

STEP 3: DETERMINE TAPING PROTOCOL AND TENSION

Once you have defined the clinical objective and considered the acuteness or chronicity of the patient, then determine what tape technique and tape tension to use. We will discuss in greater detail now the difference in techniques and tension and how it affects clinical outcomes for your patients.

FUNCTIONAL TAPING TECHNIQUES

Functional Tape is applied based on treatment goals. The variables in tape application include the amount of pre-stretch applied to the tape, position of the area to be taped, and the treatment goals (pain reduction, subcutaneous blood flow, improved muscle function) (Yasukawa, Patel, & Sisung, 2006).

When the purpose is to support injured tissue, adhesive, non-stretch (rigid) sports tape is generally most appropriate. This is applied without tension, as the tape is already rigid.

Rigid tape is made of zinc oxide which can irritate the skin without an underlay. It is very adhesive, and may be painful to remove. With the use of rigid tape, con-sider that the patient's range of motion will be restricted. Restricted range of motion in any joint may lead to compensation patterns in other posture quadrants of the body. This is an important consideration from the point of view of a Posture Expert. An acute injury may have a chronic impact of postural compensation patterns.

Functional Tape is made of acrylic, is flexible, and adheres the best to the first thing it touches. It will lose stickiness after touching the first surface it is exposed to. Flexible tapes can be worn in the shower and will remain adhesive to the skin. Although there are many examples of flexible, functional tape, the original is Kinesio tape. We will discuss Kinesio tape and the other brands at the end of this module.

A taping technique that combines rigid and flexible tape is called Specific Proprioceptive Rehabilitation Tape (SPRT). In this technique the Posture Expert will place the flexible tape first as the underlay, then utilize a rigid tape over the top with a fold to increase tension. A full demonstration will be shown in Module 4 of how to apply the tape in this taping technique.

The purpose of SPRT is to offload tissue tension to improve function. To decide where and when to use this tape, you want to manually test the direction of tissue tension and see how the patient responds. They should feel immediate relief when the skin is pulled in the proper direction. When you see that the patient is experiencing pain relief, you want to tape in that direction to reproduce pain relief.

TAPE TENSION

Kinesio tape, which again is a flexible tape, has many different functions, which we have discussed. It is very important to understand that the reason why Kinesio Tape has so many different functions is because the functions of the tape are determined by the amount of tension that the tape has.

When the tape has negative tape tension to 0% tension, the objective of this application is to reduce muscle spasm and to inhibit neural activity. When the tape is applied with negative tape tension, the Posture Expert should see convolutions of the skin under the tape. When convolutions are present it creates areas of high and low pressure. This type of tape tension would be used in chronic low back pain cases for example.

Tape with 0% to 10% tension is used to objectively achieve a reduction of swelling and muscle spasms. The objective results are an improvement in lymph and vascular flow, and an inhibition of neural activity at the site of the muscle spasm if a spasm is present. Negative tape tension, up to 10% tape tension is indicated for patients with acutely injured tissues.

When the objective goal of taping is lymphatic or edema drainage, the tape tension will be approximately 10%. The tape will stimu-

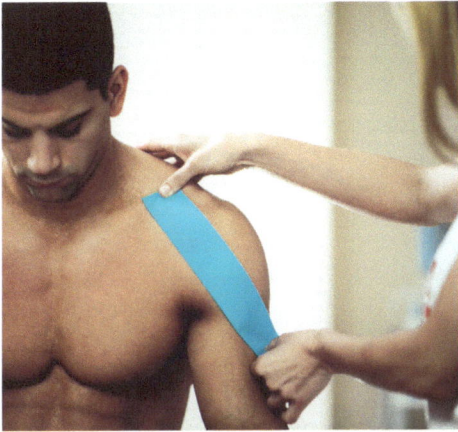

ADVANCED POSTURE TAPING PROTOCOLS

As this course is centered on Posture Taping, the clinical objective of Posture Taping is to reduce specific postural distortion patterns in combination with your regular treatment plans for patients. The improvement of posture falls within the tape tension category of 10%-50%. When applying Posture Tape, it is recommended to apply the tape with a tension of 25%. Tape at this tension, approximately 25%, will remain adhesive to the patient's skin for a longer amount of time than tape with a high amount of tension.

Patients who utilize Posture Tape should experience an immediate result in which they claim they feel "it working," or they "feel straighter" or "more upright." If the tape is applied to the cervical spine for reduction of forward head posture, the Posture Expert should see an immediate reduction of forward head posture when the tape is applied. If the tape is applied to the scapulae for reduction of anterior shoulder displacement, the patient should feel that their shoulders are back and the Posture Expert should see a change.

If there is no reported change from the patient and the Posture Expert does not see any immediate changes, then the tape should be removed and reapplied to a different postural distortion pattern, or the tension should be adjusted. Utilize the patient's feedback as important information helping you, the Posture Expert, to make objective changes with your patients.

If the patient doesn't feel anything with the application of Kinesio tape, the Posture Expert can also utilize the SPRT technique for a more profound sensation. With the utilization of the tabs when applying the tape, the pull of the tape will fee more significant to the patient.

Posture Taping is in the category of "Posture Habit Re-education." Again, the American Posture Institute recommends a three-component system for the complete correction of postural distortion patterns. These three components include: spinal alignment, posture rehabilitation, and posture habit re-education.

As Posture Taping is utilized for posture habit re-education, the patient should feel the tape making a difference in their structure immediately after it is applied. This is important, because the tape is utilized as a trigger for the patient to re-educate their postural habits. When they can feel better posture, they will be prompted to maintain this better postural position during their activities of daily living and occupational job requirements.

late Meissener's Corpuscles and lifts upper dermal layers of the skin creating space for lymphatic drainage and blood flow between the fascia and the muscle, reducing swelling and edema. This process also decompresses the sensory nerves at the site of the tape application.

Tape tension of 10%-50% is utilized to increase muscle tone by facilitating muscle firing and coordination. With up-regulated activity at the site of tape application, the body becomes more aware of the tissue, increasing proprioception. The clinical objectives of this tape tension are to increase neural activity for improved proprioception and to increase muscle tone. This taping tension will be utilized for non-acute patients to improve postural presentation, proprioception, and performance.

Tension above 50% (from 50-100%) is utilized for therapeutic pain relief. The purpose of applying tape with this amount of tension is to offload painful tissue while simultaneously increasing range of motion.

For patients with high amounts of pain, it is recommended to apply the tape with 70-80% tension. It is worth noting, that there has been no shown benefit to increase tension above 80%. In fact is not recommended to apply tape with a tension of over 80% as it may cause skin irritation.

ACUTE PATIENTS

CHRONIC PATIENTS

SUPORTIVE TAPE

CASE PRESENTATION:
- Hypermobile
  - Forward Head Posture

CLINICAL OBJECTIVE:
- Stabilize

TAPE TENSION:
- 0%-10%

EDEMA/LYMPH DRAINAGE

CASE PRESENTATION:
- Swelling, Edema

CLINICAL OBJECTIVE:
- Reduce Edema

TAPE TENSION:
- 0%

SPASMODIC TAPE

CASE PRESENTATION:
- Acute Injury

CLINICAL OBJECTIVE:
- Reduce Muscle Spasm

TAPE TENSION:
- 0%-10%

POSTURE TAPE

CASE PRESENTATION:
- Postural Distortion Patterns
  - Forward Head Posture
  - Anterior Shoulder Displacement
  - Anterior / Posterior Pelvic Tilt

CLINICAL OBJECTIVE:
- Correct Postural Distortion Patterns
- Posture Habit Re-Education

TAPE TENSION:
- 25%

THERAPEUTIC TAPE

CASE PRESENTATION:
- Chronic Pain

CLINICAL OBJECTIVE:
- Decease Pain

TAPE TENSION:
- SPRT Technique:
  - To offload painful tissues
- High Tension Tape
  - To decrease pain

PROPRIOCEPTIVE TAPE

CASE PRESENTATION:
- Functional Deficiency
  - Decreased ROM
  - Muscle Test
  - Palpation

CLINICAL OBJECTIVE:
- Increase proprioception of compromised tissue

TAPE TENSION:
- 10-50%

POSTURE TAPING ANALYSIS FLOWCHART

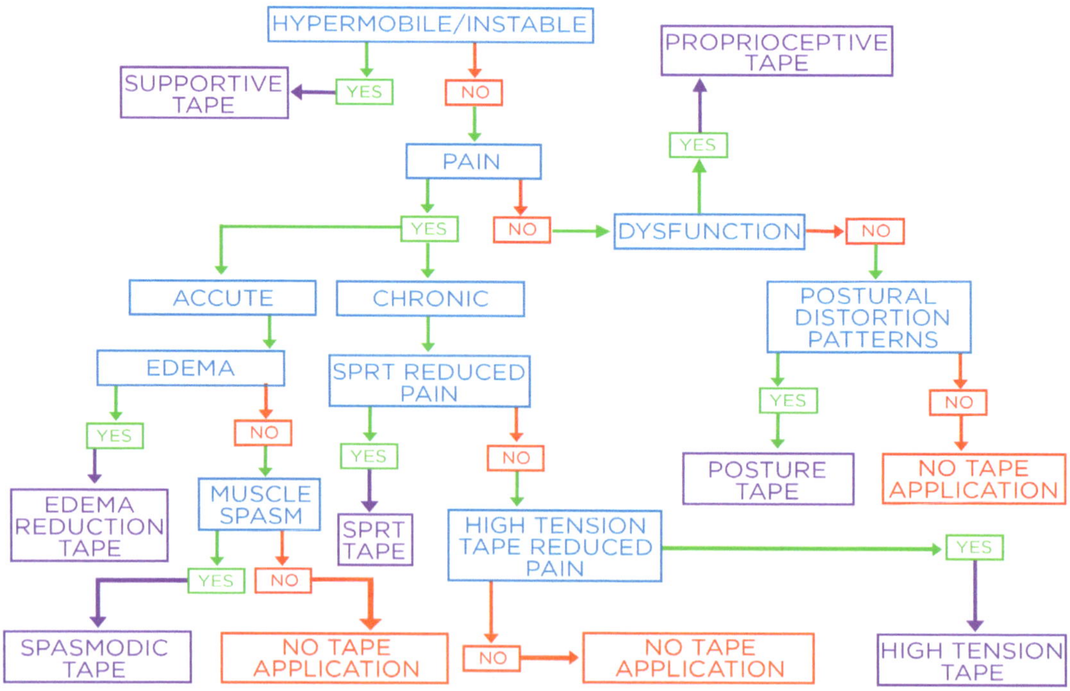

CASE PRESENTATION EXAMPLES

Let's consider specific case presentations of patients who presented to our clinic. We will go through the three-step process to determine what type of tape will be the most beneficial to their care.

PATIENT #1

The first patient is Johnny. Johnny, age 51 had been coming in as a patient for 9 weeks. Johnny sought postural correction care for the chronic pain that he felt at the base of his neck and across both shoulders. As Johnny described it, "I feel like I have a ton of bricks pushing on my neck. It kills me at work."

His treatment plan at week 9 required one in--office postural correction treatment and posture rehabilitation session per week. In addition to the in-office care, he was instructed to do daily at-home postural rehabilitation exercises.

The results of his first re-evaluation at the 6th week of care demonstrated significant objective improvements in his postural presentation. The forward head posture that he originally presented with was dramatically reduced, he had developed core strength to support proper lumbopelvic posture, and his shoulders demonstrated a decrease in anterior displacement.

Although objective results determined improvement of Johnny's postural design, his pain only diminished slightly. His pain level on the first examination was 7 out of 10. On the re-evaluation 6 weeks later, he still demonstrated a pain level of 5 out of 10. Johnny was content to see objective changes on his posture image and commented that after beginning care he feels "much straighter and lighter, but my neck pain is still killing me at work."

Recognizing the patient's frustration, at week 9 of his treatment plan Johnny began utilizing Posture Tape for therapeutic relief of the lower cervical spine and bilateral trapezius muscles.

"I feel really good," said Johnny immediately after the tape was applied to his neck and upper back. "I feel like the tape supports my neck and takes the pressure off my shoulders," he said.

How did we make this clinical decision?

Step number 1 is to determine the desired clinical outcome. In this case, the desired outcome was therapeutic relief. He presented with localized chronic pain of posture quadrant 1. He was showing objective postural correction changes with his treatment protocol, but his pain level was still high.

Step number 2 is to determine whether or not the patient was acute or chronic. Johnny was in a state of chronic pain from chronic postural distortion patterns.

Step number 3 is to determine what type of tape technique to use with what degree of tension. To obtain the clinical objective of pain relief, we decided to use Functional Tape with a tape tension of 70-80%. The purpose of applying tape with this amount of tension is to offload painful tissue without restricting their range of motion.

We decided to use High Tension Tape with Johnny as we don't recommend the utilization of SPRT for posture quadrant 1 – so this option was immediately eliminated. The pre--test and post-test to ensure that this was the appropriate clinical decision was to ask him the pain level pre and post application. He said the pain was instantly reduced, so we know it was a good clinical decision.

PATIENT #2

Now meet patient number two. At 16 years old Alexandra was experiencing excruciating headaches on average 4 days per week, and she had some lower back pain that came and went. Her headaches would usually come in the afternoon, making half of her school day absolutely miserable. Alexandra tried to pay attention in class, but the more she tried to concentrate the more her head would throb.

Alexandra's posture images and case presentation were a classic example of Text Neck. Not only was Alexandra suffering from the symptomatic consequences of poor postural design, the objective results demonstrated significant forward head posture and an increased lumbar lordosis for a 16 year old.

Because Alexandra's postural collapse was evident during certain activities, it was necessary to change her postural habits. From the moment she began her postural correction program she was given posture habit re-education recommendations to prevent postural collapse at school and while texting or using her Ipad.

At her re-evaluation, Alexandra demonstrated objective and subjective improvements. The postural presentation of her cervical spine and lumbar spine had improved in comparison to her original posture images. Plus she felt much better! She hardly ever had headaches anymore. Everything seemed to be progressing along great.

It wasn't until Alexandra's mother mentioned that she wasn't adhering to her posture habit re-education plan that we considered to use Posture Tape with her. As her mother stated, she still has bad posture when looking at her phone and while studying. Wanting to get full improvement and prevent the headaches from coming back, we decided to use Posture Tape as a means of posture habit re-education with Alexandra.

How was this clinical decision made?

Step number 1 is to determine the desired clinical outcome. The patient demonstrated subjective and objective clinical improvements without the use of Postural Tape. The only thing that was not improving was the change in her habits. The specific goal of Posture Tape for Alexandra was to improve her posture habits, specifically to prevent postural collapse of her cervical and lumbar spine.

Step number 2 is to determine whether or not the patient was acute or chronic. Alexandra was a chronic patient.

Step number 3 is to determine what type of tape technique to use with what degree of tension. For the objective of posture habit re-education, it was decided to use

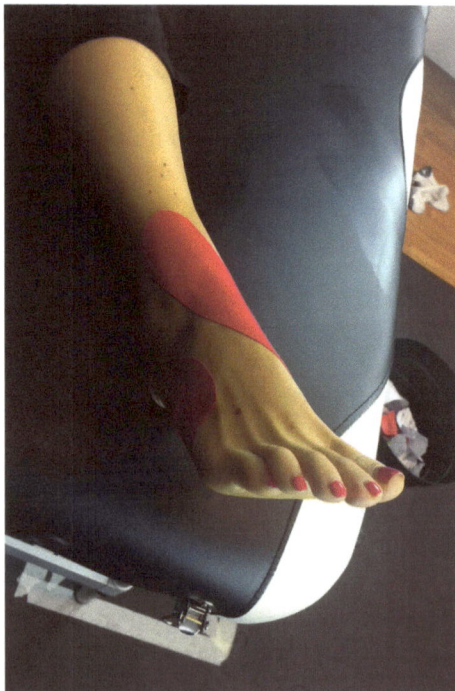

Posture Tape with a tape tension of 25%. The purpose of applying tape with this amount of tension is to up-regulate activity at the site of tape application, making the body more aware of the tissue, and increasing proprioception of the taped areas.

We utilized the full Posture Tape protocol with her as she demonstrated postural distortion patterns of the lumbar and cervical spine. The pre and post--test was to ask the patient if she felt more upright with the Posture Tape. She said she did, and stated that it was more comfortable to have good posture than to slouch. We know we made the right decision with her.

PATIENT #3

And now we have Marco, patient number 3. At 29 years old Marco is a competitive triathlete, a good one. As Marco put it, he feels strong and healthy, but was told he would compete better if came to the American Posture Institute. He was referred by one of the professional football players who had experienced significant dynamic postural correction. Improved sports performance was Marco's motivating factor to do a treatment plan of postural correction.

On Marco's re-evaluation he demonstrated toe out foot flare on his right foot and mentioned that he frequently rolled his right ankle while trail running. We tested his gait; Marco was instructed to use the JBit Medpro for gait correction, in addition to Posture Taping of his right ankle to improve ankle proprioception.

Step number 1 of this clinical decision making process was to determine the desired clinical outcome. With Marco, the objective was to improve the dysfunction causing his gait instability by increasing proprioception of the ankle joint.

Step number 2 was to consider his clinical presentation. Marco is a patient with chronic ankle instability. Had he just sprained his ankle yesterday he would be an acute patient, but this was not the case. He suffered from the chronic consequences of ankle instability.

Step number 3 was to determine what tape technique to use and what tension to use to achieve the desired clinical objective. We used Proprioceptive Tape with Marco at a tension of 30% to improve proprioception of the joint complex. Minimal tension was used to ensure that range of motion was not restricted while Marco was training.

The pre tests were to evaluate range of motion, muscle testing, and palpable muscle tonicity. There was weakness of the muscle test, the clinical objective was to facilitate the tissue surrounding the ankle.

Each of these three patients responded very well to the use of Functional Tape, all for different clinical reasons. When utilized under the correct circumstances, taping is an effective tool for subjective, objective, and performance-based outcomes. Utilize the three-step protocol with your patients to determine what the most effective taping strategy will be for them.

CLINICAL APPLICATION OF POSTURE TAPE

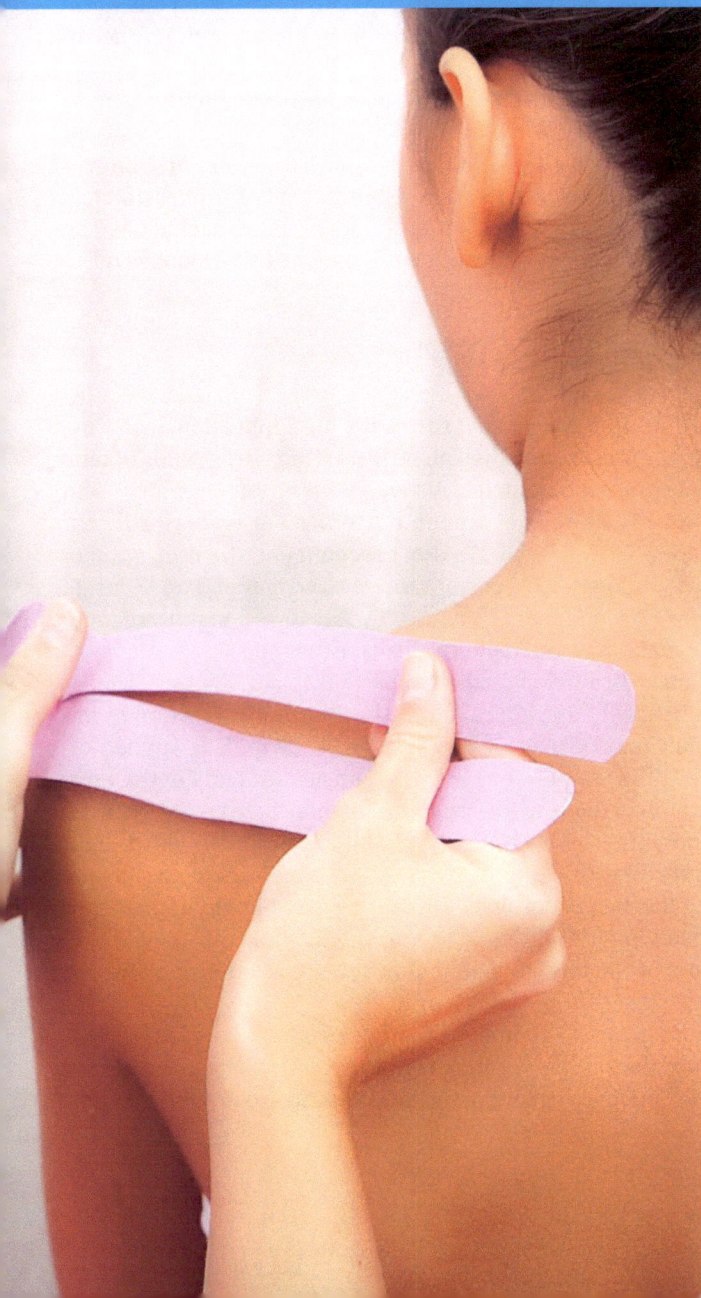

Welcome to Module 4! Now you have all the tools you need to determine which patients need Functional Tape, what kind of tape, and at what tape tension. In Module 4 you will learn specific taping techniques that you can utilize with your patients.

There are multiple things to consider when applying the tape. For example, how to prepare the patient, how to cut the Functional Tape, and how to find the desired level of tension. All of that will also be covered in this module. Then we will look at strategies of how to implement Functional Taping in your clinic. We want it to be quick and efficient for you, yet precise and patient centered.

Then we will discuss how to apply each type of Functional Tape discussed in Module 3 to the posture System. We will provide examples of each type of taping protocol within each posture quadrant. We will provide you with a lot of examples. The most important thing, however, is to understand the process of determining what taping protocol to use. Once that is decided, consider how to apply the tape with accurate tension.

Once you understand these concepts you can essentially apply tape to any tissue of the body – following sound clinical guidelines. Now let's get to work.

SPECIFIC EXPERT PROTOCOLS

With the recent popularity of the utilization of Kinesio Tape, there are so many generic protocols out there. You can simply google "Kinesio Tape for the neck" and you will get a ton of images, videos, and blogs. You can watch the YouTube video and learn how to do a protocol that looks professional, and will seem like it will work with your patients. So many of your colleagues will do this. They will apply this YouTube recommended protocol without any reason of why and without having any clinical pre or post-test. Some of their patients will feel better, and some won't.

This is not good enough for you, you are an expert.

When you provide expert level care, expect predictable, objective, outcomes. If you don't know how to test and re-test, then it is not objective enough. Experts know what they are doing and why they are doing it. Utilize the Clinical Analysis Map that we went through in Module 3 to guide you to proper clinical decision-making of when and how to apply functional tape with your patients.

EXPERT APPLICATION

Apply tape to clean skin that is ideally free of hair. Make sure the patient does not apply lotion or cream to the area where the tape will be applied. Never apply the tape directly to areas of the skin that are irritated or cut.

Functional Tape will stick to the first thing that it touches. When applying the tape on patients, do not touch the tape, or it will be less adhesive on your patient's skin. To effectively apply tape for therapeutic relief of high tension tape without touching it, pull back the layer of paper on the back of the tape at the mid point of where you will be applying it. Contact the tape to the skin, then stick the tape to the skin one side at a time, slowly peeling off the back paper layer as you go.

For longer pieces of tape that are used in all other applications than high tension therapeutic tape that we just discussed where you apply from the center point of the tape, you will apply the anchor piece first. The anchor piece has no stretch, will be rounded at each end, and is at least 1 inch long. Apply this piece first by laying it down and not touching the back. Then you can stretch the rest of the tape besides the anchor points for desired application.

Do not try to reposition the tape once it has been applied. Have a clear path of where the tape will be applied before unpeeling it. The tape should be pre-measured to ensure that it is long enough to span across the targeted tissues. To measure the area, make the measurements before the tape has been cut and before peeling back the paper. You can touch the tape directly to the body part that it will be applied before peeling it away. Also take into consideration what tension you will be using. This will make a difference of your measurement.

Once the tape has been applied, rub the surface of the tape to ensure that it is fully stuck to the skin. Apply a moderate amount of pressure and rub along the tape lengthwise. In the first hour it bonds to the outer layer of the skin. After that, it lasts approximately 3-5 days depending upon the patient's individual epithelial life. The epithelial life determines how often the patient's skin sloughs off.

FUNCTIONAL TAPE STRIPS

There are multiple ways to cut the strips for application, including the I strip, the Y strip, and the Fan strips. With many brands of tape you can buy pre-cut tape strips. Although this is not necessary – and honestly we utilize rolls of tape in our office – it is more efficient for utilization of your time. We don't recommend the utilization of pre-cut, "do it yourself" types of tape. We recommend an accurate clinical analysis leading the Posture Expert to rational protocol of when to use the tape and when not to use the tape.

The I Strip is a normal cut of tape that looks like this. The "I" Strip can be used for: pain relief and mechanical correction of improper movement patterns. To apply an "I" Strip, it is applied directly over the area of injury or pain. The anchor ends of the tape, approximately 1 inch from each end, should be applied with no stretch, while the center of the tape should be applied with a light to moderate stretch depending on the treatment objective. When the taping has been completed, the taped area should appear convoluted, showing the lifting action of the tape on the skin. Round the corners of the tape to help it stay attached to the skin without peeling off.

The Y Strip is an I strip with a cut down the center lengthwise. The anchor piece is left without a cut in order to adhere the tape to the skin. Round each corner of the tape. Y strips go around the belly of the muscle and can be used for: facilitating the activation of a weak muscle to help it contract more effectively, to inhibit the activation of an overused or injured muscle to protect it and help it recover, for mechanical correction of unsafe or inefficient movement patterns, for educing pain and inflammation, and for softening scar tissue, reducing adhesions and pitting, making scars softer, flatter and more pliable.

To apply the "Y" strip, the base should be applied slightly above or below the belly of the muscle being taped. The two tails of the "Y" are applied along the outer borders of the muscle belly.

The Fan Strip is a Y strip that has then been cut in half again. As always, round each of the corners of the tape. Apply the anchor piece first, and then fan the strips outward. This application is utilized specifically for the reduction of edema, swelling, and lymphatic drainage. It can be applied directly over contusions to reduce the amount of visible bruising.

HOW TO GET DESIRED TAPE TENSION

When the tape is on the roll it has approximately 10% tension. This is due to the white strip on the back to protect the adhesive and the rolling of the tape. To get negative tension you have to relax the tape when taken off the roll so there is no stretch to it. It should look "flimsy" and "swoop" down in the center.

For application of tape with negative to 0% tape tension, the Posture Expert must pre-stretch the tissue before applying the tape. The pre-stretch of the tissue allows for convolutions to be present when the tape is applied over the pre-stretched tissue. When applying tape at this tension, convolutions should be seen immediately after the application is complete.

Applying tape at suggested tensions can be quite subjective. To prevent in-consistencies of application follow a procedure when applying the tape. To determine what percent of tension you are using, you want to first stretch the tape to 100%, then relax it back from 100% to the desired tension.

TAPING APPLICATIONS OF THE POSTURE SYSTEM

Now we will demonstrate how to apply tape to the Posture System to achieve your desired clinical result. We will go through each type of taping protocol for each Posture Quadrant. Please utilize the shown methods as examples. It is important to understand the clinical analysis and how to the different taping protocols. Once you understand these two concepts you can apply the tape to any part of the body, it is not limited to the examples provided here.

Consider the following examples that are specifically used with the acute patient group.

SUPPORTIVE TAPE

Supportive tape will not be shown in this course. This is used for instable or hypermobile patients, for example, patients with an acute sprained ankle or hyperextended elbow. For these patients you goal is to restrict range of motion and you will use restrictive tape to do this. Again, the reason we are not demonstrating it is because we don't work with athletes who have a new acute injury, there are other healthcare professionals for this. We see patients a few weeks later. Even when Dr. Mark is working on the sidelines at professional sports games he is not the person to tape ankles with restrictive tape before the game, the physiotherapist does this. As a Posture Expert for the team he is interested in increasing range of motion, proprioception, alignment, and mobility of the athletes, not restricting it.

EDEMA/LYMPH DRAINAGE TAPING PROTOCOL

When applying tape for the purpose of lymphatic drainage or to reduce edema, the anchors are applied on the lymph nodes, and then apply a fan application to drain the lymph away from the nodes. The tape is applied with a tension of 0%. To achieve 0% tension, elongate the area for which the tape is being applied and pre-stretch the tissue. Once the tape is applied, you will see convolutions of the tape on the skin.

Please note: this taping protocol will not be recommended for posture quadrant 1. When performing any type of tape to the cervical spine or back, it is important to apply tape bilaterally (at different tensions), but always bilaterally.

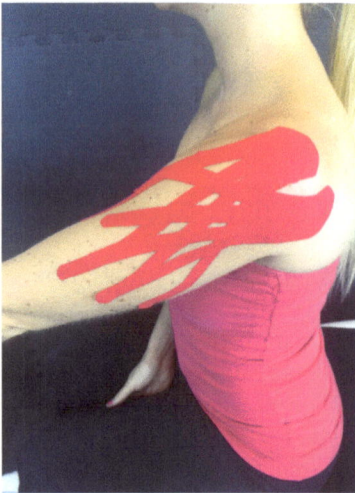

POSTURE QUADRANT 2:

Application of tape from the shoulder down the arm

Clinical Objective: To reduce edema

Case Presentation: Acute edema

Tape Tension: Tape applied at 0% tension with pre-stretch of the tissue

Pre and Post Test: No pre or post test for this application

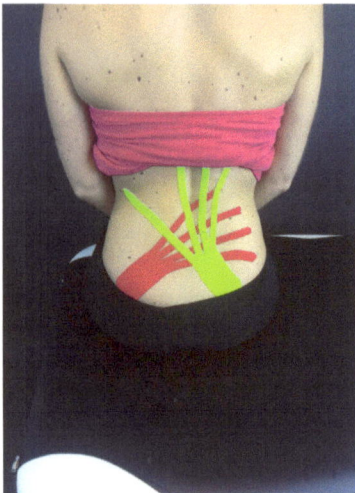

POSTURE QUADRANT 3:

Application of tape to the lower back

Clinical Objective: To reduce edema

Case Presentation: Acute edema

Tape Tension: Tape applied at 0% tension with pre-stretch of the tissue

Pre and Post Test: No pre or post test for this application

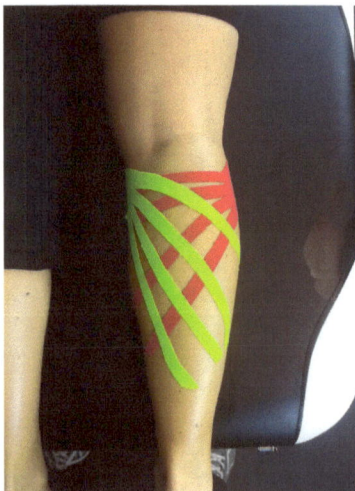

POSTURE QUADRANT 4:

Application of tape to the calf

Clinical Objective: To reduce edema

Case Presentation: Acute edema

Tape Tension: Tape applied at 0% tension with pre-stretch of the tissue

Pre and Post Test: No pre or post test for this application

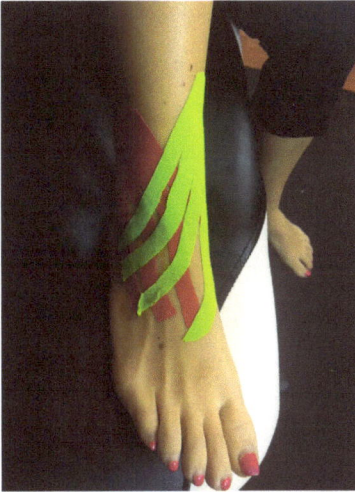

POSTURE QUADRANT 4:

Application of tape to the foot

Clinical Objective: To reduce edema

Case Presentation: Acute edema

Tape Tension: Tape applied at 0% tension with pre-stretch of the tissue

Pre and Post Test: No pre or post test for this application

SPASMODIC TAPING PROTOCOL

This type of taping protocol is to reduce muscle spasm of acute patients. The tape tension is negative to 0%, and is applied from insertion to origin. To achieve negative tension, you must pre-stretch the tissue before applying the tape. You will see convolutions after the tape is applied. The pre and post application tape for this type of taping is to ask the patient how they feel. Do they feel less tension in their muscle with the tape on?

Below you will find an example of how to apply the tape to one muscle of each posture quadrant. You can utilize this protocol of taping for any muscle that demonstrates acute muscle spasm.

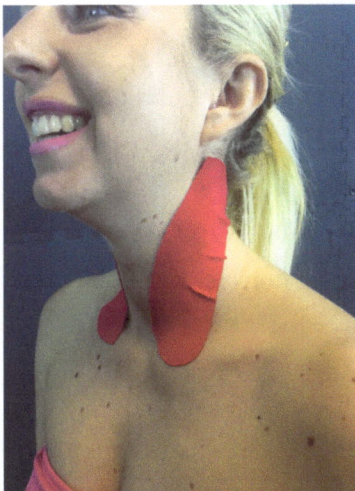

POSTURE QUADRANT 1:

Application of tape to the sternocleidomastoid musculature

Clinical Objective: To reduce acute muscle spasm

Case Presentation: Acute muscle spasm

Tape Tension: Tape applied at 0% tension with pre-stretch of the tissue

Pre and Post Test: Ask the patient if they feel relief of muscle spasm

Expert Tip: Apply the tape to each side of the cervical spine. Apply to the side with muscle spasm with 0% tension. Apply to the opposite side at "Tape Off Tension"

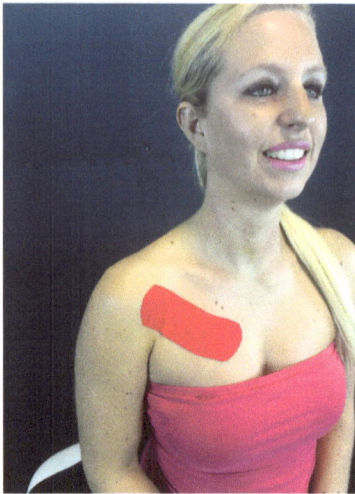

POSTURE QUADRANT 2:

Application of tape to the pectoralis musculature

Clinical Objective: To reduce acute muscle spasm

Case Presentation: Acute muscle spasm

Tape Tension: Tape applied at 0% tension with pre-stretch of the tissue

Pre and Post Test: Ask the patient if they feel relief of muscle spasm

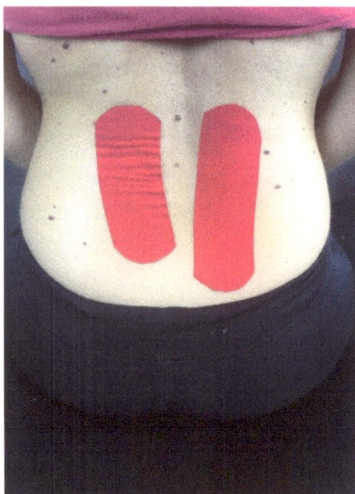

POSTURE QUADRANT 3:

Application of tape to the lumbar erector spinae musculature

Clinical Objective: To reduce acute muscle spasm

Case Presentation: Acute muscle spasm

Tape Tension: Tape applied at 0% tension with pre-stretch of the tissue

Pre and Post Test: Ask the patient if they feel relief of muscle spasm

Expert Tip: Apply the tape to each side of the cervical spine. Apply to the side with muscle spasm with 0% tension. Apply to the opposite side at "Tape Off Tension"

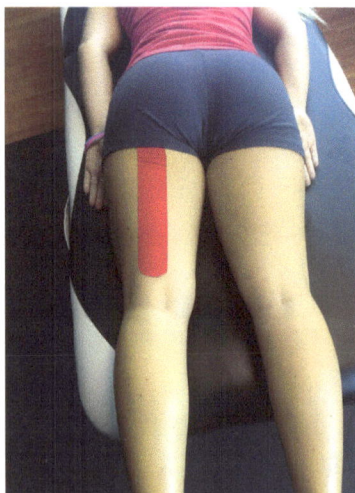

POSTURE QUADRANT 4:

Application of tape to the hamstring musculature

Clinical Objective: To reduce acute muscle spasm

Case Presentation: Acute muscle spasm

Tape Tension: Tape applied at 0% tension with pre-stretch of the tissue

Pre and Post Test: Ask the patient if they feel relief of muscle spasm

POSTURE TAPE PROTOCOL

The purpose of posture tape is to put the patient in the appropriate position, then tape the area of the postural distortion pattern at 25-30%. You will have the patient contract their musculature during the application to maintain the proper postural position.

For the purpose of posture habit re-education we recommend doing a general posture taping protocol that will be appropriate for the postural distortion patters of the lower back, of anterior displacement of the shoulders, and for forward head posture. Start by using the full protocol. Then, to avoid the patient becoming reliant on the tape to maintain proper posture, do regressions of the Posture Tape. For example: do the full protocol for two applications, on the third application don't apply tape to the lower back, then on the next application don't apply the tape to the cervical spine, then eliminate the shoulder tape as well.

You can also apply the tape to the individual posture quadrants to correct local postural distortion patterns. For the application of tape to the neck with the intention of correcting forward head posture, for example, have the patient retract their neck into proper posture, then apply the tape.

The pre and post test for Posture Tape is that the patient should feel straighter or more upright immediately after the tape is applied. Ask the patient what they feel after the application has been applied. Also perform a pre and post posture evaluation to evaluate for postural changes.

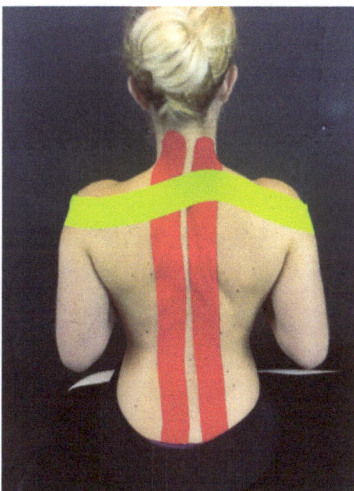

FULL POSTURE TAPE PROTOCOL:

Application of tape to posture quadrants 1- 3

Clinical Objective: To improve posture through posture habit re-education

Case Presentation: Chronic postural distortion patterns

Tape Tension: Tape applied at 25% tension with pre-stretch of the tissue

Pre and Post Test: Ask the patient if they feel like they have better posture. Evaluate their postural presentation pre and post tape application

Expert Tip: Apply the tape to each side of the cervical spine. Apply to the side with muscle spasm with 0% tension. Apply to the opposite side at "Tape Off Tension"

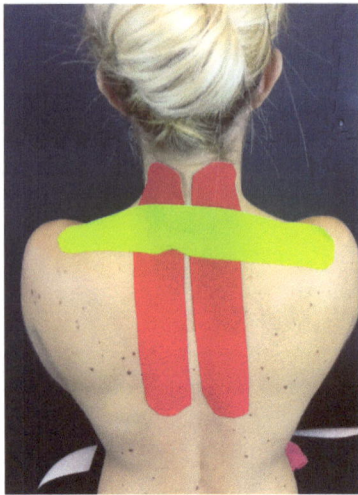

POSTURE QUADRANT 1:

Application of tape for forward head posture

Clinical Objective: To improve posture through posture habit re-education

Case Presentation: Chronic postural distortion patterns

Tape Tension: Tape applied at 25% tension with pre-stretch of the tissue

Pre and Post Test: Ask the patient if they feel like they have better posture. Evaluate their postural presentation pre and post tape application

Expert Tip: Apply the tape to each side of the cervical spine. Apply to the side with muscle spasm with 0% tension. Apply to the opposite side at "Tape Off Tension"

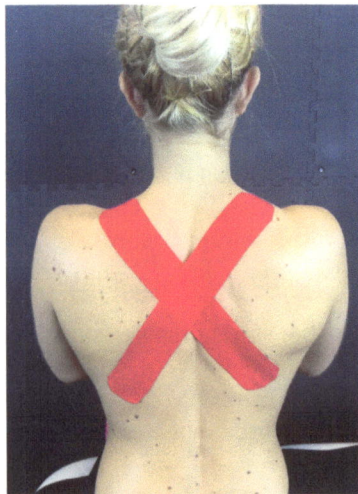

POSTURE QUADRANT 2:

Application of tape for anterior shoulder displacement

Clinical Objective: To improve posture through posture habit re-education

Case Presentation: Chronic postural distortion patterns

Tape Tension: Tape applied at 25% tension with pre-stretch of the tissue

Pre and Post Test: Ask the patient if they feel like they have better posture. Evaluate their postural presentation pre and post tape application

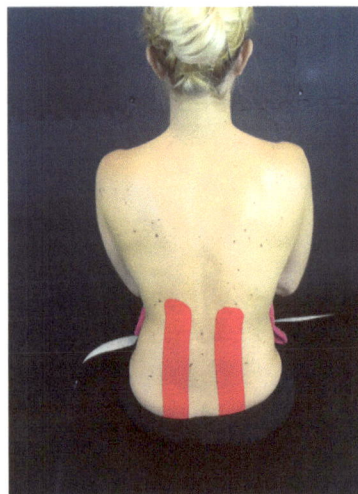

POSTURE QUADRANT 3:

Application of tape for lumbopelvic postural distortion patterns

Clinical Objective: To improve posture through posture habit re-education

Case Presentation: Chronic postural distortion patterns

Tape Tension: Tape applied at 25% tension with pre-stretch of the tissue

Pre and Post Test: Ask the patient if they feel like they have better posture. Evaluate their postural presentation pre and post tape application

Expert Tip: Apply the tape to each side of the cervical spine. Apply to the side with muscle spasm with 0% tension. Apply to the opposite side at "Tape Off Tension"

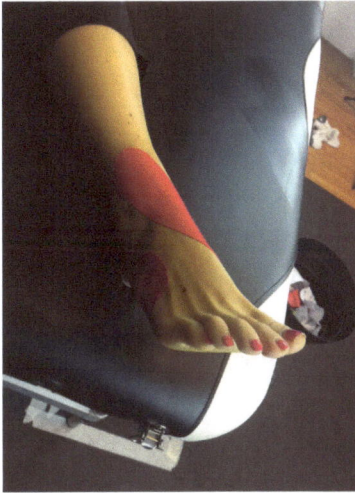

Application of tape for pronation of the foot

Clinical Objective: To improve posture through posture habit re-education

Case Presentation: Chronic postural distortion patterns

Tape Tension: Tape applied at 25% tension with pre-stretch of the tissue

Pre and Post Test: Ask the patient if they feel like they have better posture. Evaluate their postural presentation pre and post tape application

PROPRIOCEPTIVE TAPE PROTOCOL

The purpose of proprioceptive tape is to improve dysfunction by inhibiting or facilitating muscles that demonstrate dysfunction. To improve dysfunction, the specific location of dysfunction needs to first be located; this is accomplished by completing three different pre-tests to localize the area of dysfunction.

The three pre-tests include: Testing range of motion of the intended area, performing muscle tests to determine for muscular weakness, and palpating the area to evaluate for hyper or hypo tonicity that needs to be facilitated or inhibited.

Once you perform these three tests and localize the level of dysfunction, then decide if the musculature needs to be facilitated or inhibited.

To facilitated the tissue, apply the tape with a tape tension of 20-50%. The patient will elongate the musculature that the tape is being applied to, and the tape is applied from origin to insertion.

To inhibit the tissue, apply the tape with a tape tension of 0%. The tissue will be pre--stretched and the tape is applied from insertion to origin.

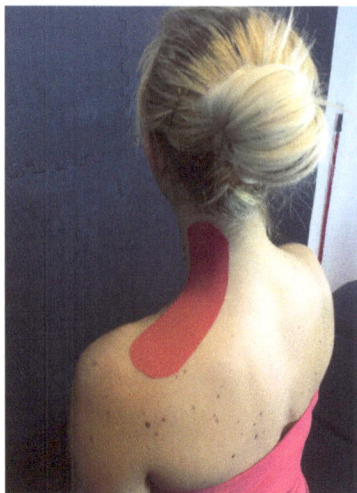

POSTURE QUADRANT 1:

Application of tape to facilitate the upper trapezius

Clinical Objective: To improve proprioception by facilitating tissue

Case Presentation: Chronic performance related dysfunction

Tape Tension: Tape applied at 20-50% tension with pre-stretch of the tissue

Pre and Post Test:

- **ROM:** to determine ROM pre and post application
- **Muscle Test:** to evaluate muscle strength pre and post application
- **Palpation:** to evaluate muscle tonicity pre and post application

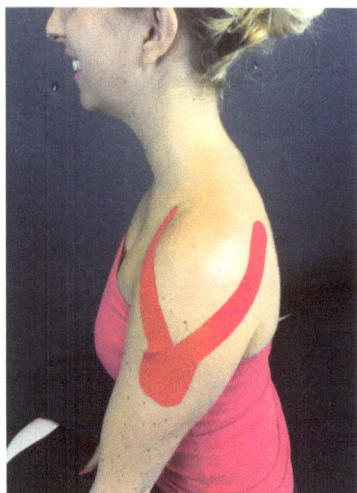

POSTURE QUADRANT 2:

Application of tape to facilitate the shoulder complex

Clinical Objective: To improve proprioception by facilitating tissue

Case Presentation: Chronic performance related dysfunction

Tape Tension: Tape applied at 20-50% tension with pre-stretch of the tissue

Pre and Post Test:

- **ROM:** to determine ROM pre and post application
- **Muscle Test:** to evaluate muscle strength pre and post application
- **Palpation:** to evaluate muscle tonicity pre and post application

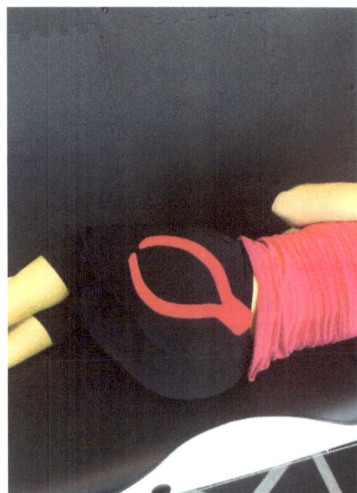

POSTURE QUADRANT 3:

Application of tape to facilitate the gluteus maximus

Clinical Objective: To improve proprioception by facilitating tissue

Case Presentation: Chronic performance related dysfunction

Tape Tension: Tape applied at 20-50% tension with pre-stretch of the tissue

Pre and Post Test:

- **ROM:** to determine ROM pre and post application
- **Muscle Test:** to evaluate muscle strength pre and post application
- **Palpation:** to evaluate muscle tonicity pre and post application

*Please note, the tape is applied over the clothing only for purposes of demonstration. It should be applied to the skin.

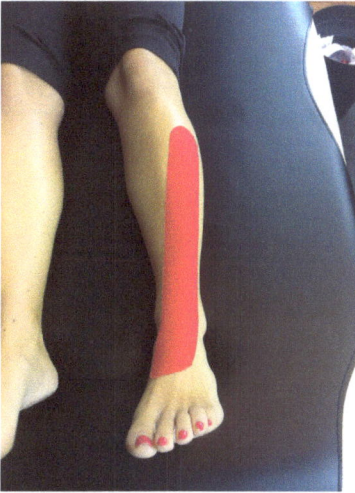

POSTURE QUADRANT 4:

Application of tape to facilitate the tibialis anterior

Clinical Objective: To improve proprioception by facilitating tissue

Case Presentation: Chronic performance related dysfunction

Tape Tension: Tape applied at 20--50% tension with pre-stretch of the tissue

Pre and Post Test:

- **ROM:** to determine ROM pre and post application
- **Muscle Test:** to evaluate muscle strength pre and post application
- **Palpation:** to evaluate muscle tonicity pre and post application

*Please note, this taping protocol is not recommended for posture quadrant 1

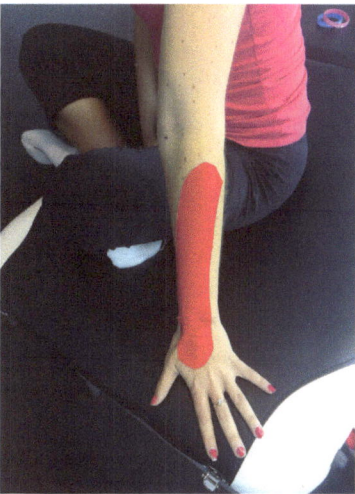

POSTURE QUADRANT 2:

Application of tape to inhibit the forearm extensor musculature

Clinical Objective: To improve proprioception by inhibiting hypertonic tissue

Case Presentation: Chronic performance related dysfunction

Tape Tension: Tape applied at 0% tension with pre-stretch of the tissue

Pre and Post Test:

- **ROM:** to determine ROM pre and post application
- **Muscle Test:** to evaluate muscle strength pre and post application
- **Palpation:** to evaluate muscle tonicity pre and post application

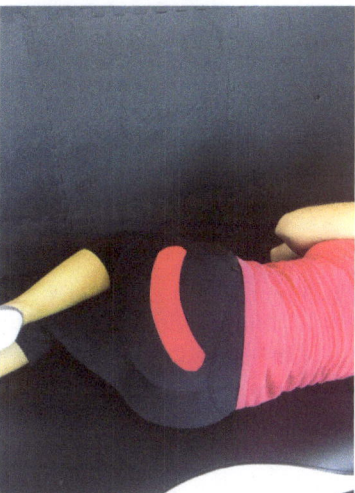

POSTURE QUADRANT 3:

Application of tape to inhibit the piriformis

Clinical Objective: To improve proprioception by inhibiting hypertonic tissue

Case Presentation: Chronic performance related dysfunction

Tape Tension: Tape applied at 0% tension with pre-stretch of the tissue

Pre and Post Test:

- **ROM:** to determine ROM pre and post application
- **Muscle Test:** to evaluate muscle strength pre and post application
- **Palpation:** to evaluate muscle tonicity pre and post application

*Please note, the tape is applied over the clothing only for purposes of demonstration. It should be applied to the skin.

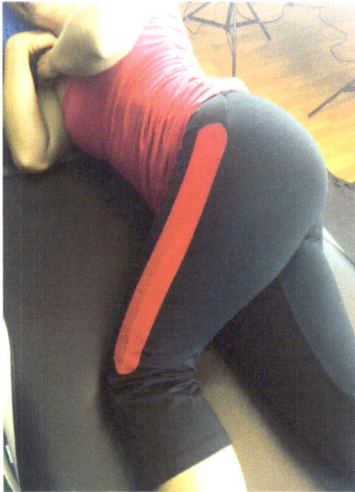

POSTURE QUADRANT 4:

Application of tape to inhibit the tensor fascia lata

Clinical Objective: To improve proprioception by inhibiting hypertonic tissue

Case Presentation: Chronic performance related dysfunction

Tape Tension: Tape applied at 0% tension with pre-stretch of the tissue

Pre and Post Test:

• **ROM:** to determine ROM pre and post application

• **Muscle Test:** to evaluate muscle strength pre and post application

• **Palpation:** to evaluate muscle tonicity pre and post application

*Please note, the tape is applied over the clothing only for purposes of demonstration. It should be applied to the skin.

THERAPEUTIC TAPE

The purpose of therapeutic tape is to off load painful tissue. When this is performed accurately, the patient should immediately feel pain relief. This will be your pre and posttest, to ask the patient how they feel after the tape is applied to the painful tissue.

There are two types of therapeutic taping. To determine which one to use, you want to test the tissue with tension in different directions to offload the tissue first. If you move the tissue in a certain direction and the patient feels less pain, then they would benefit from specific proprioceptive rehabilitation taping or the SPRT taping protocol applied in that direction.

SPRT TAPE:

SPRT is Specific Proprioceptive Rehabilitation Taping. With this type of taping protocol you will utilize two forms of tape, restrictive tape and functional tape. The functional tape is an underlay to protect the skin, and the restrictive tape is the overlay. To achieve more tension, you will make tabs on the tape, then place your finger at the base of the tab, apply a second piece of Restrictive Tape and tape over your finger to increase tension and pull the tissue in the direction that reduces pressure. The pre and post test is to determine for pain reduction.

HIGH TENSION TAPE:

If tissue stress in different directions does not reduce pain, you will use the High Tension Tape protocol. This is used with the goal of eliminating pain. You will localize the area of pain and apply an I strip with a minimum of 50% tension and a maximum of 80% tension. For the majority of patients, tape will be applied at 70-80% tension for maximal benefit. The tape is applied from origin to insertion. The pre and post test is to determine for pain reduction.

*Please note, this taping protocol is not recommended for posture quadrant 1

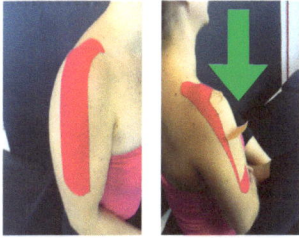

Place finger here and tape over it

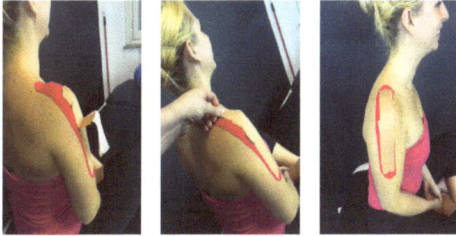

POSTURE QUADRANT 2:

Application of SPRT tape to the deltoid musculature

Clinical Objective: To reduce pain by offloading tissue

Case Presentation: Chronic pain

Tape Tension: Tape applied at with high tension due to tabs for increased tissue tension

Pre and Post Test: to ask the patient if they feel reduced pain with the application of tape

Expert Tip: Make tab, place finger at the base of the tab, then with the other hand tape over the tab, pulling the tape in the direction that offloads the tissue and reduces the pain

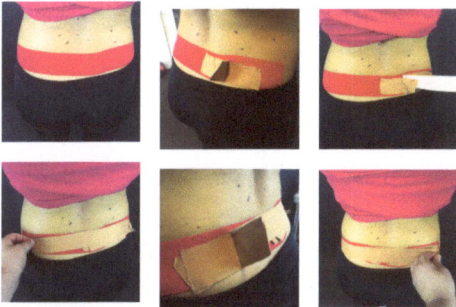

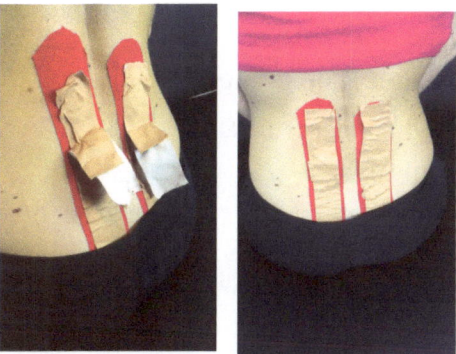

POSTURE QUADRANT 3:

Application of SPRT tape to the sacroiliac joints bilaterally

Clinical Objective: To reduce pain by offloading tissue

Case Presentation: Chronic pain

Tape Tension: Tape applied at with high tension due to tabs for increased tissue tension

Pre and Post Test: to ask the patient if they feel reduced pain with the application of tape

Expert Tip: Make tab, place finger at the base of the tab, then with the other hand tape over the tab, pulling the tape in the direction that offloads the tissue and reduces the pain

POSTURE QUADRANT 3:

Application of SPRT tape to the lumbar erector spinae musculature

Clinical Objective: To reduce pain by offloading tissue

Case Presentation: Chronic pain

Tape Tension: Tape applied at with high tension due to tabs for increased tissue tension

Pre and Post Test: to ask the patient if they feel reduced pain with the application of tape

Expert Tip: Make tab, place finger at the base of the tab, then with the other hand tape over the tab, pulling the tape in the direction that offloads the tissue and reduces the pain

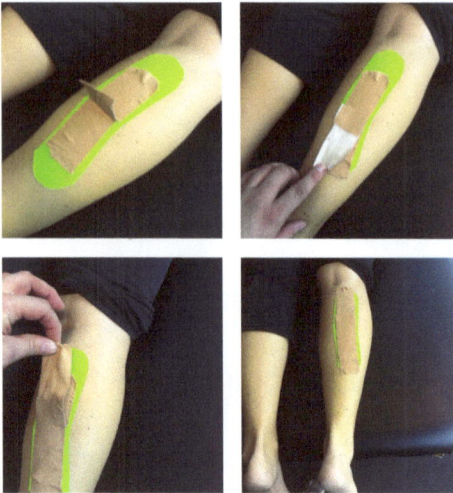

POSTURE QUADRANT 4:

Application of SPRT tape to the calf musculature

Clinical Objective: To reduce pain by offloading tissue

Case Presentation: Chronic pain

Tape Tension: Tape applied at with high tension due to tabs for increased tissue tension

Pre and Post Test: to ask the patient if they feel reduced pain with the application of tape

Expert Tip: Make tab, place finger at the base of the tab, then with the other hand tape over the tab, pulling the tape in the direction that offloads the tissue and reduces the pain

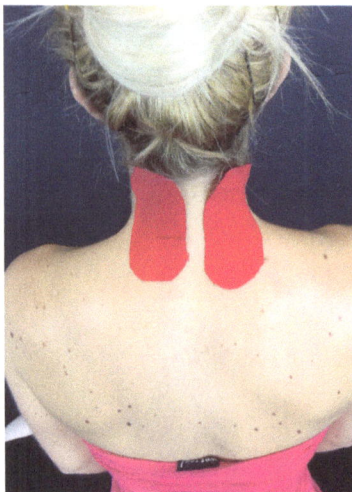

POSTURE QUADRANT 1:

Application of High Tension Tape to the trapezius muscles bilaterally

Clinical Objective: Immediate pain relief

Case Presentation: Chronic pain

Tape Tension: Tape applied at 70-80% tension with pre-stretch of the tissue

Pre and Post Test: to ask the patient if they feel reduced pain with the application of tape

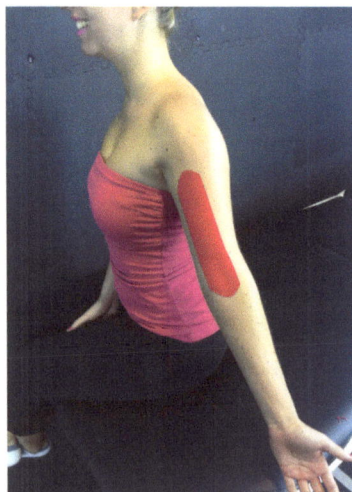

POSTURE QUADRANT 2:

Application of High Tension Tape to the bicep

Clinical Objective: Immediate pain relief

Case Presentation: Chronic pain

Tape Tension: Tape applied at 70-80% tension with pre-stretch of the tissue

Pre and Post Test: to ask the patient if they feel reduced pain with the application of tape

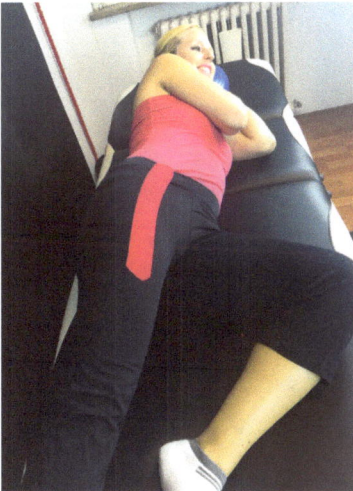

POSTURE QUADRANT 3:

pplication of tape High Tension Tape to the iliopsoas

Clinical Objective: Immediate pain relief

Case Presentation: Chronic pain

Tape Tension: Tape applied at 70-80% tension with pre-stretch of the tissue

Pre and Post Test: to ask the patient if they feel reduced pain with the application of tape

*Please note, the tape is applied over the clothing only for purposes of demonstration. It should be applied to the skin.

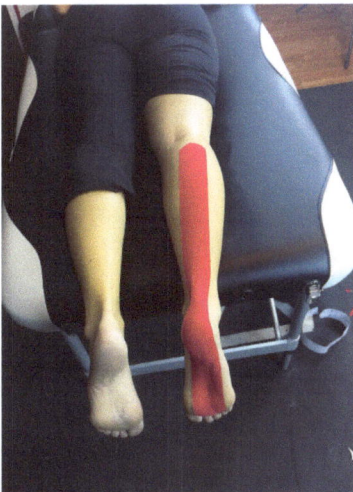

POSTURE QUADRANT 4:

Application of High Tension Tape of the Achille's tendon

Clinical Objective: Immediate pain relief

Case Presentation: Chronic pain

Tape Tension: Tape applied at 70-80% tension with pre-stretch of the tissue

Pre and Post Test: to ask the patient if they feel reduced pain with the application of tape

Bonus Section

CONDITION SPECIFIC TAPING PROTOCOLS

In this section you are provided with a quick reference for some of the most common case presentations that will come to your office. As always, the recommendation is to utilize the Clinical Analysis Flowchart to determine the location of pain/dysfunction/or postural distortion.

When utilizing these taping protocols, still determine your clinical objective and apply the appropriate amount of tape tension. If you want to facilitate proprioception utilize tape tension of 25-50%. If your goal is to reduce pain, utilize tape tension of 70-80%.

Follow the same application instructions that were provided earlier in the course.

Lateral Epicondylitis Tape Application

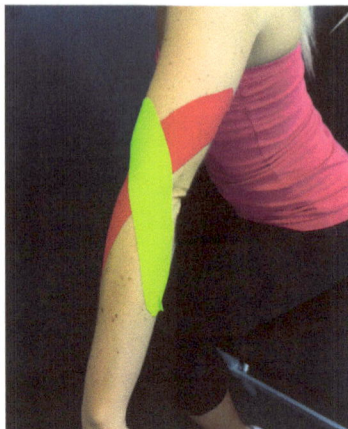

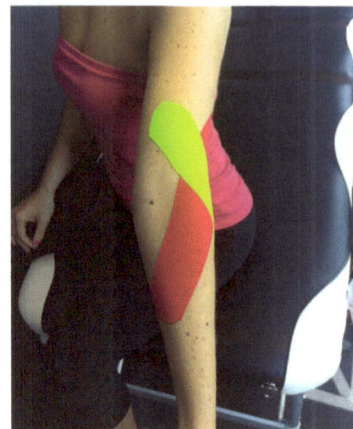

Medial Epicondylitis Tape Application

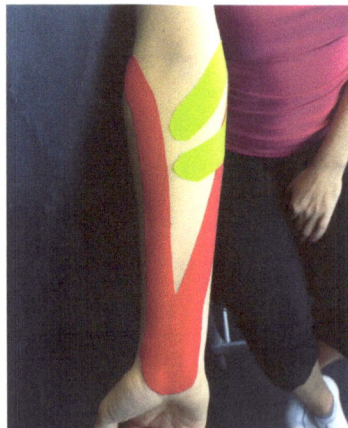

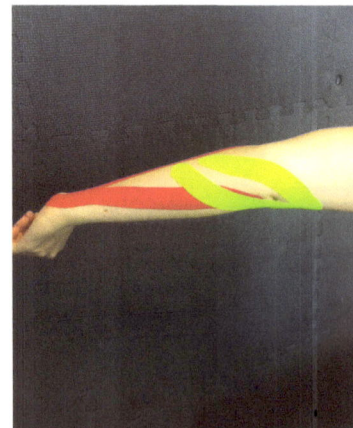

Carpal Tunnel Syndrome Tape Application

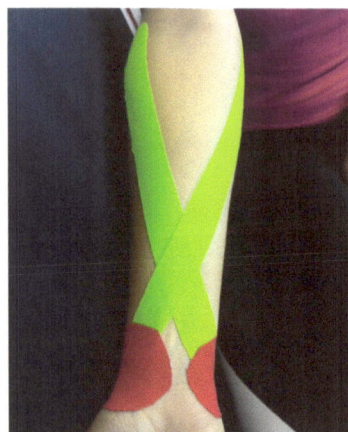

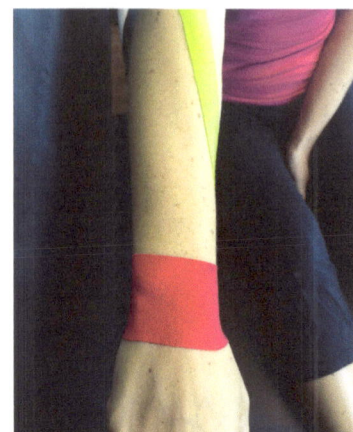

Shoulder Capsulitis Syndrome Tape Application

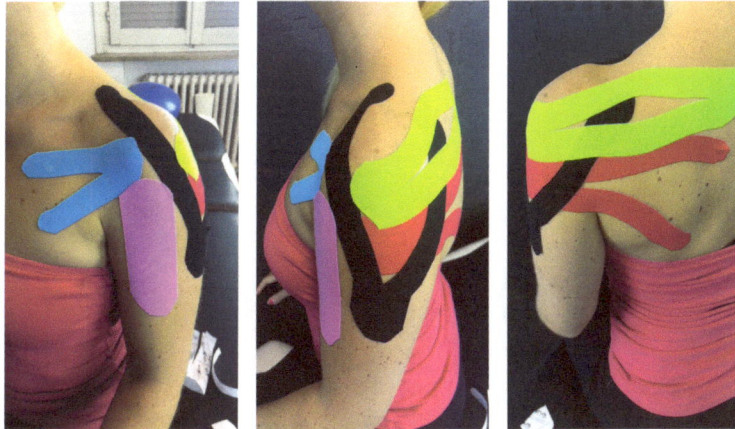

Knee Osteoarthritis Tape Application

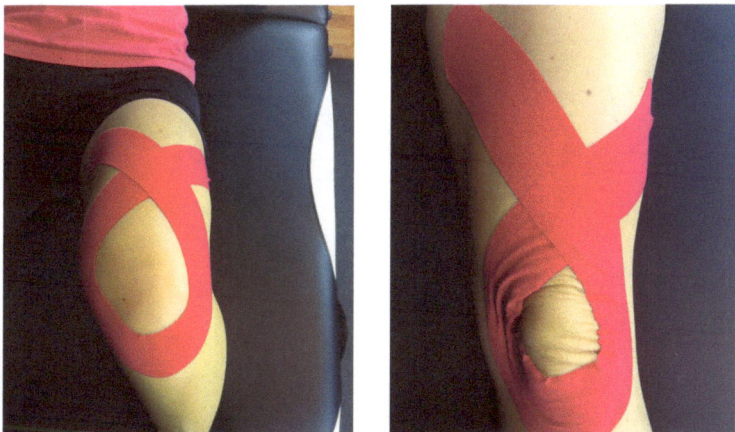

Fat Pad Bursa Tape Application

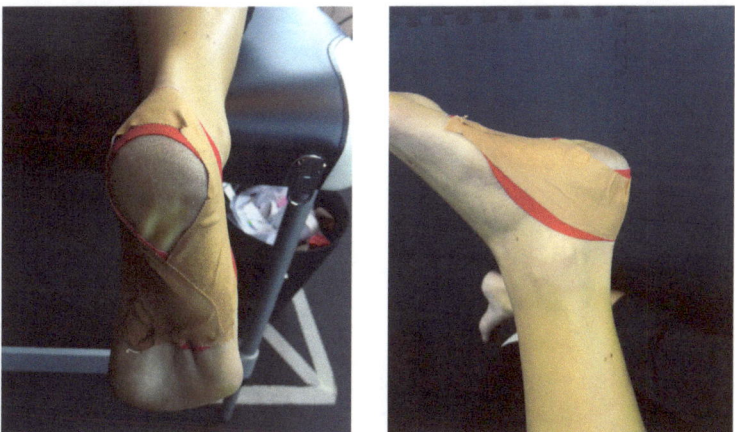

Plantar Fascitis Tape Application

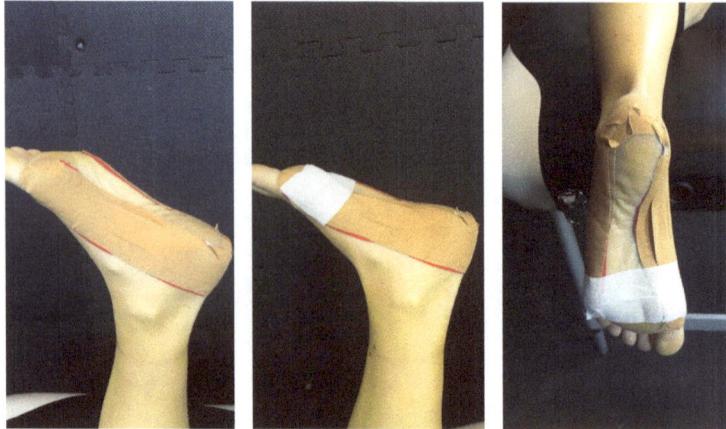

Shin Splints Tape Application

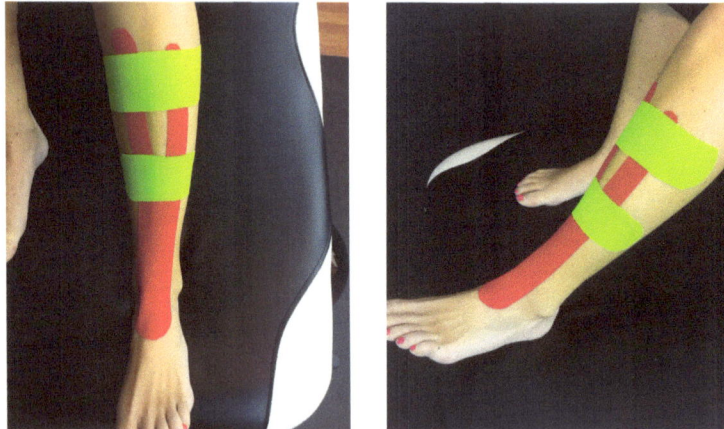

Hammer Toe Tape Application

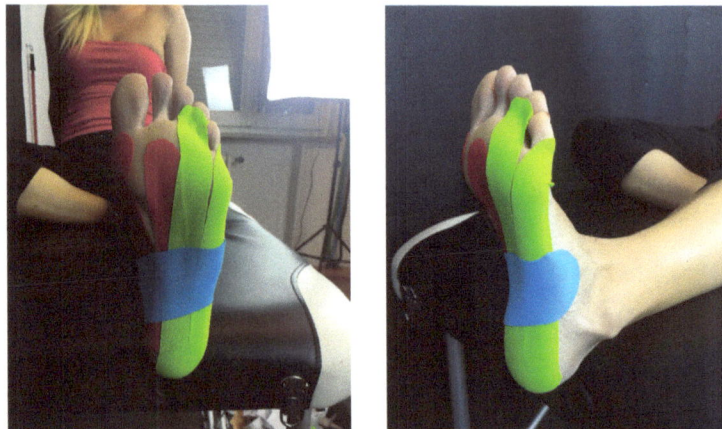

Thumb Hypermobilization Tape Application

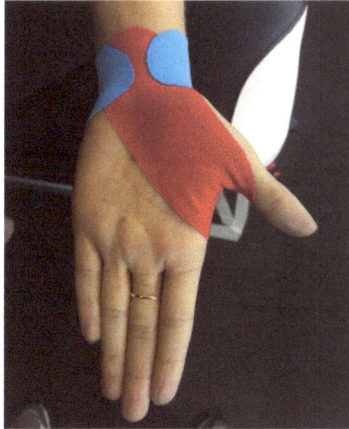

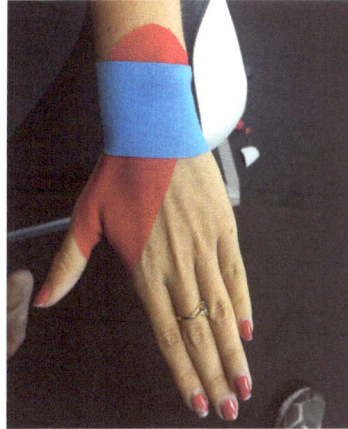

Indigestion Tape Application

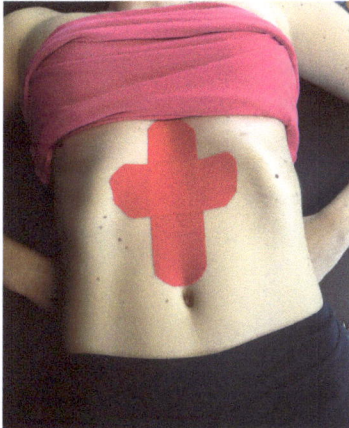

IMPLEMENTATION OF FUNCTIONAL TAPE IN CLINICAL PRACTICE

At the American Posture Institute, we want to set you up for success. We always say, "Your Success is Our Priority." To be set up for success, there are multiple things to consider when you begin implementing Functional Tape into your practice.

First, you need to get the materials you need. What's really exciting about the implementation of Functional Tape in your practice, is that it requires such minimal equipment. The initial investment is very minimal for the returns you can receive.

The materials you will need include: a pair of sharp scissors that will not stick to the adhesive glue. This is a must when cutting the tape.

To prepare the patient for the application, you will need cleaning supplies, such as alcohol to remove perspiration, oil, lotion, etc. from the surface of the skin. There is also pre--made cleaner that you can apply directly to the skin and wipe off.

Now you need to decide what type of tape to use in your office and to make the order. We utilize, and recommend that others do too, the large rolls of tape. This is the most cost efficient, and doesn't run out as quickly. Although getting pre-cut tape would save time, it is much more expensive, and is not patient specific with the measurements.

You have what you need, now you need to tell your patients – and potential new patients! With any new program or item that you want to feature in your clinic, you should always do a value added campaign to educate your patients.

Internal marketing and educational opportunities include: posting information on your white boards, making flyers and placing them in places where the patient will see them while waiting for treatment or performing an exercise, talking about it to your patients during table talk,

emailing your contacts, and of course doing a Posture Workshop all about Functional Taping. Posture Workshops are the most effective.

For external marketing, invite potential new patients to come to the posture workshop. Also utilize Facebook marketing outreach and fill your social media channels with information relevant to taping and how it has helped others just like them. Testimonies and patient stories are strong social proof.

While you are gathering the materials and preparing the marketing, you also need to educate your staff. Your staff will often have more interaction with the patient than you do. They need to be able to answer questions, and be knowledgeable about the tape.

You can also train them to do the full application if this is within the laws and regulations of your state. You decide what kind of taping protocol to do. Train them to pre--cut the tape, clean the skin, and explain about the tape to the patient, so you can walk in the room and make the application. Or, if your state or country allows it, the staff member can go forth with the application.

Once you begin using the tape you should also charge your patients appropriately. You can charge for the tape itself, from 10 -15$ or for the full application including your time: anywhere from $15-50.

When deciding what to charge, consider the difference of you applying the tape versus your staff, and charge accordingly.

When to use the tape? This is completely up to you, however, we recommend having a plan in place. With our patients, we begin utilizing tape after the first re-- evaluation. At this point we have a clear idea of their postural distortion patterns, dysfunction if it's still present, and if they still have pain or not.

We then continue to apply the tape until the clinical objective is met. You don't want the patient to be reliant on the tape, but you want to utilize it enough to achieve the desired clinical result. If not, there is not point in applying the tape at all.

There are many opportunities available with the usage of Functional Tape! You have all the information you need, so get to work, and have fun doing it.

Posture By Design, Not By Circumstance

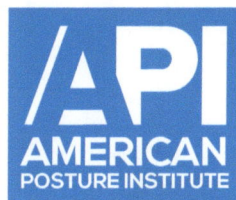

/API
AMERICAN
POSTURE INSTITUTE

REFERENCES

Bragg, R., Macmahon, J., & Overom, E., et al (2002) Failure and fatigue characteristics of adhesive athletic tape. Med Sci Sports Exerc 34(3):403–410.

Briem, K., Eythorsdottir, H., Magnusdottir, R., Palmarsson, R., Runarsdottir, R., & Syeinsson, T. (2011) Effects of Kinesio Tape Compared With Nonelastic Sports Tape and the Untaped Ankle During a Sudden Inversion Perturbation in Male Athletes. *Journal of Orthopaedic & Sports Physical Therapy*, 41(5) 328–335.

Castro-Sanchez, A., Lara-Palomo, I., Penarrocha, G., Fernandez-Sanchez, M., Sanchez-Labraca, N., & Arroyo-Morales, M. (2012) Kinesio Taping reduces disability and pain slightly in chronic non-specific low back pain: a randomised trial. *Journal of Physiotherapy*, 58(2) 89-95.

Cepeda, J., Fishweicher, A., Gleeson, M., Greenwood, S., & Motyka-Miller, C. (2008) Does Kinesio Taping of the abdominal muscles improve the supine-to-sit transition in children with hypotonia? http://www.kinesiotaping.com/kinesio-taping-forabdominal-muscles-to-improve-the-supine-to-sit-transition-inchildren.php

Chang, H., Chou, K., Lin, J., Lin, C., & Wang, C. (2010) Immediate effect of forearm Kinesio taping on maximal grip strength and force sense in healthy collegiate athletes. *Physical Therapy in Sport*, 11 122-127.

Clark, K. (2014) Use of Kinesio Taping as an Adjunct to Positioning. *Clinical Corner*. 2015.5 40-43.

Cole, A., McGrath, M., Harrington, S., Padua, D., Rucinski, T., & Prentice, W. (2013) Scapular Bracing and Alteration of Posture and Muscle Activity in Overhead Athletes With Poor Posture. *Journal of Athletic Training*, 48(1) 12-24.

Dawood, R., Katabei, O., Nasef, S., Battarjee, K., & Abdelraouf, O. (2013) Effectiveness of Kinesio Taping versus Cervical Traction on Mechanical Neck Dysfunction. *International Journal of Therapies and Rehabilitation Research*, 2(2).

DiMatteo, M. (1995) Patient adherence to pharmacotherapy: the importance of effective communication. *Formulary*, 30(10) 596-8, 601-2, 605.

Detsky, A. (2011) What Patients Really Want. *JAMA*, 306(22).

Elshemy, S. & Bettecha, K. (2013) Kinesio Taping Versus Proprioceptive Training on Dynamic Position Sense of the Ankle and Eversion to Inversion Strength Ratios in Children with Functional Ankle Instability. *Med. J. Cairo Univ.*, 81(2) 61-68.

Fayson, S., Needle, A., & Kaminski, T. (2013) The Effects of Ankle Kinesio® Taping on Ankle Stiffness and Dynamic Balance. *Research in Sports Medicine*, 21(3) 204-216.

Fejer R, Kyvik KO, Hartvigsen J. (2006) The prevalence of neck pain in the world population: a systematic critical review of the literature. *Eur Spine J.*, 15 834–848.

Gardner, B., Lally, P., & Wardle, J. (2012) Making health habitual: the psychology of 'habit-formation' and general practice. *The British Journal of General Practice*, 62(605) 664-666.

Gomez-Soriano, J., Abian-Vicen, J., Aparicio-Garcia, C., Ruiz-Lazaro, P., Simon-Martinez, C., Bravo-Esteman, E., & Fernandez-Rodriguez, G. (2013) The effects of Kinesio taping on muscle tone in healthy subjects: A doubleblind, placebo-controlled crossover trial. *Manual Therapy*, 19 131-136.

Gonzalez-Iglesias, J., Fernandez-De-Las-Penas, C., Cleland, J., Huijbregts, P., & Gutierrez-Vega, M. (2009) Short-Term Effects of Cervical Kinesio Taping on Pain and Cervical Range of Motion in Patients With Acute Whiplash Injury: A Randomized Clinical Trial. *Journal of Orthopedic and Sports Physical Therapy*, 39(7) 515-521.

Halseth, T., McChesney, J., DeBeliso, M., Vaughn, R., & Lien, J. (2004) The Effects of Kinesio™ Taping on Proprioception at the Ankle. *Journal of Sports Science and Medicine*, 3(1) 1-7.

Han, J., Lee, J., & Yoon, C. (2015) The mechanical effect of kinesiology tape on rounded shoulder posture in seated male workers: a single-blinded randomized controlled pilot study. *Physiotherapy Theory and Practice*, 31(2) 120-5.

Hsu, Y., Chen, W., Lin, H., Wang, W., & Shih, Y (2009) The effects of taping on scapular kinematics and muscle performance in baseball players with shoulder impingement syndrome. *J Electromyogr Kinesiol*, 19 1092–1099.

Huang, C., Hsieh, T., Lu, S., & Su, F. (2011) Effect of the Kinesio tape to muscle activity and vertical jump performance in healthy inactive people. *BioMedical Engineering OnLine*, 10(70).

Jaraczewska, E. & Long, C. (2006) Kinesio® Taping in Stroke: Improving Functional Use of the Upper Extremity in Hemiplegia. *Topics in Stroke Rehabilitation*, 13(3) 31-42.

Jin, J., Sklar, G., Oh, V., & Li, S. (2008) Factors affecting therapeutic compliance: A review from the patient's perspective. *Ther Clin Risk Manag.*, 4(1) 269-286.

Kase K. 1994. Illustrated Kinesio Taping®, 3rd Ed., Ken'I Kai, To-kyo, pp.90--91.

Kase, K., Tatsuyuki, H., & Tomoko, O. (1996) Development of Kinesio tape. Kinesio Taping Perfect Manual. Kinesio Taping Association.

Kaya, E., Zinnuroglu, M., & Tugeu (2011) Kinesio taping compared to physical therapy modalities for the treatment of shoulder impingement syndrome. *Clin Rheumatol* (2011) 30 201-207.

Kelly, R., Zyanski, S., & Alemagno, S. (1991) Prediction of motivation and behavior change following health promotion: Role of health beliefs, social support, and self-efficacy. *Social Science and Medicine*, 32(3) 311-320.

Ladislav Pyšný, Jana Pyšná, Dominika Petrů. 2015. Kinesio Taping Use in Prevention of Sports Injuries During Teaching of Physical Education and Sport. Procedia - Social and Behavioral Sciences 186, 618.

Lee, J., & Yoo, W. (2011) The Mechanical Effect of Anterior Pelvic Tilt Taping on Slump Sitting by Seated Workers. *Industrial Health*, 49, 403-409.

Lee, J., Yoo, W., & Hwang--Bo, G. (2011). The Immediate Effect of Anterior Pelvic Tilt Taping on Pelvic Inclination. *Journal of Physical Therapy Science*, 23 201-203.

Lemos, T., Albino, A., Matheus, J., & Barbosa, A. (2014) The Effect of Kinesio Taping in Forward Bending of the Lumbar Spine. *Journal of Physical Therapy Science*, 26(9) 1371-1375.

Lin, J., Hung, C., & Yang, P. (2011) The effects of scapular taping on electromyographic muscle activity and proprioception feedback in healthy shoulders. *Journal of Orthopaedic Research*, 29(1) 53--57.

Luque-Suarez, A., Noguero, G., Baron-Lopez, F., Manzanares, M., Hush, J., & Hancock, M. (2014) Effects of kinesiotaping on foot posture in participants with pronated foot: A quasi-randomised, double-blind study. *Physiotherapy*, 100 36-40.

Mostafavifar, M., Wertz, J., & Borchers, J. (2015) A Systematic Review of the Effectiveness of Kinesio Taping for Musculoskeletal Injury. *The Physician and Sportsmedicine*, 40(4).

Mostert-Wentzel, K., Swart, J., Masenyetse, L., Sihlali, B., Cilliers, R., Clarke, L., Martiz, J., Pinsloo, E., & Steenkamp, L. (2012) Effect of kinesio taping on explosive muscle power of gluteus maximus of male athletes. *South African Journal of Sports Medicine*, 24(3) 75-80.

Nakajima, M. & Baldridge, C. (2013) THE EFFECT OF KINESIO® TAPE ON VERTICAL JUMP AND DYNAMIC POSTURAL CONTROL. *Int J Sports Phys Ther*, 8(4) 393-406.

Neal D, Wood , Labrecque J, & Lally P. (2012) How do habits guide behavior? Perceived and actual triggers of habits in daily life. *J Exp Soc Psychol.*, 48 492-498.

Physio Advisor "Posture Taping" http://www.physioadvisor.com.au/11768450/posture--taping--improving--posture-- physioadvisor.htm.

Saavedra-Hernandez, M., Castro-Sanchez, A., Arroyo-Morales, M., Cleland, J., Lara-Polom, A., & Fernandez-De-Las-Penas, C. (2012) Short-Term Effects of Kinesio Taping Versus Cervical Thrust Manipulation in Patients With Mechanical Neck Pain: A Randomized Clinical Trial. *Journal of Orthopaedic & Sports Physical Therapy*, 42(8) 724-730.

Sackett, D. (1976) Compliance with therapeutic regimens. Baltimore: *Johns Hopkins University Press*, 1–6.

Shields, C., Needle, A., Rose, W., Swanik, C., & Kaminski, T. (2013) Effect of Elastic Taping on Postural Control Deficits in Subjects With Healthy Ankles, Copers, and Individuals With Functional Ankle Instability. *American Orthopaedic Foot and Ankle Society* 1-9.

Simsek, T., Turkucuoglu, B., Cokal, N., Ustunbas, G., Simsek, I. (2011) The effects of Kinesio taping on sitting posture, functional independence and gross motor function in children with cerebral palsy. *Disability and Rehabilitation*, 33(21–22): 2058–2063.

Slupik, A., Dwornik, M., Biatoszewski, D., & Zych, E. (2007) Effect of Kinesio Taping on bioelectrical activity of vastus medialis muscle. Preliminary report. *Ortopedia, Traumatologia, Rehabilitacja*, 9(6) 644-651.

Smykla, A. et al. (2013) Effect of Kinesiology Taping on Breast Cancer-Related Lymphedema: A Randomized Single-Blind Controlled Pilot Study. *BioMed Research International*.

Strachan, D. & Sandstrom, U. (2015) Total Taping: A Comprehensive, Conceptual Approach to Taping in the Clinical Setting. *Total Taping Seminar*.

Taradaj, J., Halski, T., Zdunczyk, M., Rajfur, J., Pasternok, M., Chmielewska, D., Piecha, M., Kwashna, K., & Plinta, V. (2014) Evaluation of the effectiveness of kinesio taping application in a patient with secondary lymphedema in breast cancer: a case report. *Prz Menopauzalny*, 13(1) 73-77.

Teutsch, C. (2003) Patient--Doctor Communication. *Med CLin N Am*, 87 1115--45.

Thedon T, et al. (2011) Degraded postural performance after muscle fatigue compensated by skin stimulation. *Gait Posture*, 33(4) 686–9.

Thelen, M., Dauber, J., & Stoneman, P. (2008) The Clinical Efficacy of Kinesio Tape for Shoulder Pain: A Randomized, Double--Blinded, Clinical Trial. *Journal of Orthopedic and Sports Physical Therapy*, 38(7) 389-95.

Tieh-Cheng Fu, A., Yu-Cheng Pei, K., & Shih-Wei Chou, Y. (2008) Effect of Kinesio taping on muscle strength in athletes–A pilot study. *Journal of Science and Medicine in Sport*, 11, 198--201.

Trotter, L. (2013) Kinesiology Tape for Postural Control. *American Journal of Clinical Chiropractic*.

Tsai, H., Jung, H., Huang, C., & Tsauro, J. (2009) Could Kinesio tape replace the bandage in decongestive lymphatic therapy for breast-cancer-related lymphedema? A pilot study. *Support Care Cancer*, 17(11) 1353-60.

Vanherzeel, M., Cingel, R., Maenhout, A., De Mey, K., & Cools, A. (2013) Does the Application of Kinesiotape Change Kinematica in Healthy Female Handball Players? *Sports Medicine*, 34 950-955.

Verplanken, B. & Wood, W. (2006) Interventions to Break and Create Consumer Habits. *Journal of Public Policy & Marketing* 25(1) 90-103.

Yasukawa, A., Patel, P. & Sisung, C. (2006) Pilot Study: Investigating the Effects of Kinesio Taping® in an Acute Pediatric Rehabilitation Setting. *The American Journal of Occupational Therapy*, 60(1) 104-110.

Yoo, W. (2013) Effect of the Neck Retraction Taping (NRT) on Forward Head Posture and the Upper Trapezius Muscle during Computer Work. *Journal of Physical Therapy Science*, 25(5) 581–582.

Yoshida, A. & Kahanov, L. (2007) The Effect of Kinesio Taping on Lower Trunk Range of Motions. *Research in Sports Medicine*, 15(2), 103-112.

PICTURE CREDITS

www.ingramcontent.com/pod-product-compliance
Lightning Source LLC
Chambersburg PA
CBHW060802270326
41926CB00002B/66